ANTI-INFLAMMATORY DIET GUIDE FOR BEGINNERS

IMPROVE YOUR HEALTH, SLOW THE AGING PROCESS, LOOK YOUNGER, LIVE LONGER

BELLA BOOKS

Copyright © 2022 Bella Book

All rights reserved.

Copyright © Bella Books 2022. All rights reserve

The content contained within this book may not be reproduced, duplicated, or transmitted without direct written permission from the author or publisher. All product and company names mentioned herein may be trademarks of their respective owners.

Under no circumstances will any blame or legal responsibility be held against the publisher or author for any damages, reparation, or monetary loss due to the information contained within this book, either directly or indirectly. You are responsible for your own choices, actions, and results.

Legal Notice: This book is copyright protected. This book is only for personal use. You cannot amend, distribute, sell, quote, or paraphrase any part, or use the content within this book, without the consent of the author or publisher.

Please note the information contained within this document is for educational and entertainment purposes only. All effort has been executed to present accurate, up-to-date, reliable, and complete information. No warranties of any kind are declared or implied. Readers acknowledge that the author is not engaging in the rendering of legal, financial, medical, or professional advice. The content within this book has been derived from various sources. Please consult a licensed professional before attempting any techniques outlined in this book. By reading this document, the reader agrees that under no circumstances are the author or publisher responsible for any losses, direct or indirect, which are incurred as a result of the use of the information contained within this document, including (but not limited to) errors, omissions, or inaccuracies.

Dedication

This book is dedicated to my grandmother, Beulah.

Table of Contents

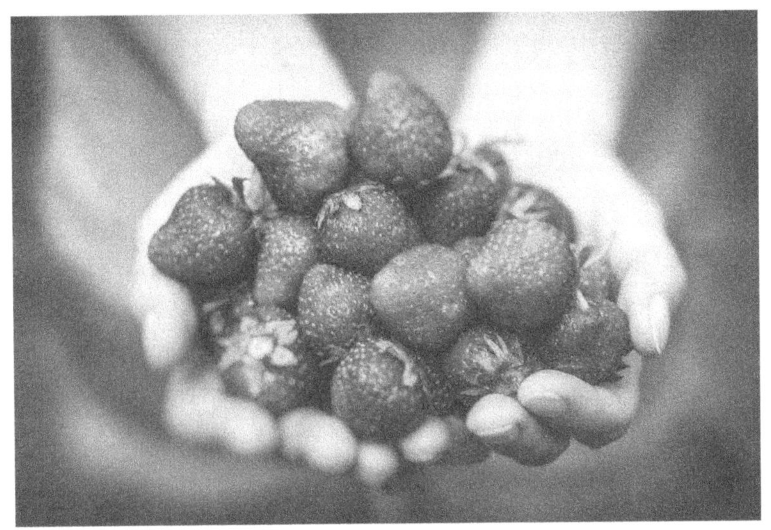

Introduction

If you have ever done any research on the Anti-Inflammatory Diet, you know that there is quite a bit of conflicting information. A diet that is really so simple seems to have become much more complicated than it needs to be. This book breaks it all down for you in a very simplistic, easy-to-understand, and implement approach.

The Anti-Inflammatory Diet is designed to replace inflammation triggering foods with delicious nutrient dense foods that fight inflammation. In this diet, what you don't eat is just as important as what you do eat. It is a lifestyle change and once you can digest that, you've got it.

Fortunately, through anti-inflammatory living, we can not only prevent future diseases from occurring but we can also reverse existing conditions and greatly improve how we feel on a daily basis. When it comes to inflammation, food is truly the best medicine.

And, when we start to view our bodies as a whole and start living an anti-inflammatory lifestyle, we see positive results from the inside out.

Understanding The Inflammation Process

Before we dive into the Anti-Inflammatory Diet, you need to have a clear understanding of the inflammatory process. As most of you probably already know, inflammation is part of our body's natural immune response. When our immune system detects an injury or invader - like a cut, sprain, bacteria, or virus, it sends inflammatory cells to the area for help. If there is an injury, the inflammatory cells will help the damaged tissue heal. If it is an invader such as a virus or bacteria, its job is to fight the invader off and get rid of it. Your white blood cells flood the area to provide protection and healing. This type of inflammation is called acute inflammation.

Chronic inflammation is totally different from acute and is thought to be the cause of several different diseases. Your body's response is the same as with acute inflammation but there isn't anything that needs healing. Your body inaccurately sends out a message that there is an issue that needs healing when it doesn't. Typically, chronic inflammation is less painful than acute inflammation but lasts for a longer amount of time and can lead to persistent inflammation.

There are several types of chronic inflammation such as Asthma, Chronic Obstructive Pulmonary Disease (COPD), Crohn's Disease, Lupus, Psoriatic Arthritis, Psoriasis, Rheumatoid Arthritis, and Ulcerative Colitis.

Common causes of chronic inflammation include:

- Autoimmune diseases, such as rheumatoid arthritis and lupus, in which the body's immune system mistakenly attacks healthy cells, causing pain, swelling, and other discomfort.
- An unresolved acute inflammation resulting from a past injury or infection.
- Prolonged exposure to certain toxins, such as industrial emissions.

In addition to autoimmune diseases, chronic inflammation is associated with several other serious health conditions. Researchers believe that chronic inflammation can trigger the disease processes for many different conditions over time.

Chronic inflammation is also linked to:

- High blood pressure
- Irritable bowel syndrome
- Psoriasis
- Alzheimer's disease
- Asthma
- Cancer
- Heart disease
- Type 2 Diabetes

Chronic inflammation does not always cause noticeable symptoms. When it does, possible symptoms of chronic inflammation may include:

- Aches and pains
- Fatigue
- Fever
- Joint pain and stiffness
- Skin rashes

When your body is in a state of chronic inflammation, it can be triggered by the foods that you eat. This is one of the reasons why an anti-inflammatory diet is so important.

Inflammation & Aging

Did you know that inflammation increases as we age? It does, it's called inflammaging. The good news is that you can reduce inflammation with just a few tweaks to your diet and lifestyle.

One of the reasons that this occurs is that as we age, the effects of unhealthy lifestyle choices take their toll. Even if you usually make the best choices regarding your overall health most of the time, no one is perfect. An unhealthy diet, stress, inactivity, smoking, and lack of sleep all play a part.

Another reason why aging causes inflammation is that as we age, our bodies tend to have more consistently elevated levels of inflammatory biochemicals. While these chemicals are good because they help our immune systems fight off infections and keep us healthy, if they are chronically elevated, they can lead to problematic things such as muscle wasting and even cancer.

There are many things that add to the inflammatory response such as highly processed foods, chronic stress, and even poor dental health. Over time, these things can weaken the body and speed up aging. This means that eating a whole food anti-inflammatory diet, getting enough sleep, exercising regularly, taking care of your teeth, and reducing or eliminating stress will all help to minimize inflammation.

Fortunately, more and more people today are becoming aware that our diets influence much more than our weight. Our health shines from the inside out. So not only is our health affected by what we eat, so is our appearance. Whoever said beauty comes from within was ahead of their time. Although that original statement had a different meaning, our appearance and how we age is affected by what we eat. Our external appearance tends to reflect our internal health. When low inflammation levels are maintained in the body, everything functions better. This in turn is reflected in our overall appearance. Research has proven that the best diet to look and feel younger is through a diet that reduces the body's inflammatory response.

Not only does this type of unfocused inflammation accelerate the aging process, it can lead to the faster onset of age-related diseases like Alzheimer's, certain cancers, cardiovascular disease, and ultimately a shorter lifespan.

The Benefits of An Anti-Inflammatory Diet

Dieticians, doctors, and specialists from around the world agree that an anti-inflammatory diet is significantly beneficial to our overall health. Nutrient dense foods contain properties known to reduce inflammation which could in turn improve health conditions, slow the aging process, and even lead to a longer life!

Foods considered anti-inflammatory are rich in vitamins, minerals, omega-3 fats, antioxidants, and other beneficial compounds. These nutrients help support your immune system so it can work better. An anti-inflammatory diet also protects your cells from damage and blocks harmful inflammatory pathways throughout your body.

People who practice anti-inflammatory diets tend to have a lower risk of developing most chronic diseases. If you already have a chronic condition, an anti-inflammatory diet can keep it from getting worse. It can also help you manage symptoms of that chronic condition.

There are many ways that your body can react to an anti-inflammatory diet. A few of the possible beneficial reactions might include:

- Less anxiety and brain fog
- More energy
- Better sleep
- Better/Clearer skin/less break out
- Weight loss
- Less bloating

- Fewer Headaches or headaches completely go away
- Lower blood pressure
- Lower cholesterol levels
- Lower blood sugar
- A decrease in muscle and joint pain
- Less overall swelling - hands & feet
- Improvement in stomach issues (gas, nausea, diarrhea, etc.)

The Basics

Fill Up On Fiber

Along with its notorious role in digestive health, fiber can combat inflammation by lowering C-reactive protein (CRP), a biomarker of inflammation found in the blood.

In addition to inflammation, fiber is also good for both digestive and heart health.

General recommendations suggest males and females should consume a minimum of 38 and 25 grams of dietary fiber daily, with adequate amounts of water/fluids.

Reduce Processed Meats

Animal meats do supply the body with protein, vitamins, and minerals, but on the anti-inflammatory diet, processed meats should be avoided or at least reduced.

Processed meats tend to be produced from meats high in saturated fats, undergo high-temperature cooking methods, and are oftentimes injected with a number of artificial flavors and preservatives.

To lessen the risk of inflammation, processed meats are recommended no more than once or twice per month.

If you are like many of us that enjoy a turkey sandwich, rather than buying packaged turkey slices, get it from the deli at your grocery store. Voila - your turkey is no longer processed. Or, start getting a healthy brand like Open Nature, for example that has no preservative, nitrates, or nitrites.

Though sodium is needed for critical body processes, too much can cause inflammation.

An additional concern relates to individuals living with rheumatoid arthritis. The medication that they are prescribed can cause the body to retain sodium more easily, consequently causing individuals to retain water and experience an increase in blood pressure.

Swap Refined Grains with Whole Grains

Refined carbs are essentially whole grains stripped away from fiber and nutrients.

Low-fiber diets and processed carbs have been linked to inflammation.

Try to make at least half of total grain consumption whole grains. Take a look at the examples below.

Examples:

Regular White Rice Risotto

Biscuits made with white flour

Regular Pasta

Barley risotto

Whole Wheat Biscuits

Whole Wheat Pasta

While following vegetarian and vegan lifestyles are based on individual preferences, plant-based foods are a primary focus in an anti-inflammatory diet.

Add more plant-based proteins into your diet. This would include beans and lentils just to name a couple, as they are also high in fiber, antioxidants and other anti-inflammatory substances.

One delicious way to do this is using beans to substitute meat. For example, instead of regular tacos, have black bean tacos.

Snack on Nuts

Nuts are rich in healthy fat and have shown to be very helpful with inflammation.

They are also rich in protein and fiber, which are dietary contributors to weight loss.

A handful of nuts, or ¼ th cup, is the recommended serving size.

Drink Alcohol in Moderation

Research suggests that moderate drinking may be advantageous to health, because of the flavonoids and antioxidants found in red wine and probiotics offered in some beer.

But, too much alcohol can cause damage to liver cells, promote inflammation, and subsequently weaken the body's immune system.

If you do drink, just remember that moderation is key. The suggested amount is one drink per day for women and 2 drinks per day for men.

Fruits and Veggies

Choose vibrant colors of fruits and vegetables to maximize nutrient content and increase fiber intake. For example, a red bell pepper would be a great choice.

The vitamin C found in citrus fruits also acts as a powerful antioxidant and can boost the immune system.

Just remember the more natural vibrant color in your diet, the better.

Olive oil is mentioned several times throughout the rest of this book for several very good reasons. It is a heart-healthy monounsaturated fat, and contains antioxidants and oleocanthal.

Oleocanthal is a phenolic compound shown to offer anti- inflammatory benefits. It is specific to olive oil, and has exhibited the same anti-inflammatory response as NSAIDs (Non-Steroidal Anti-inflammatory Drugs - like ibuprofen). But olive oil is a natural anti-inflammatory and unlike NSAIDS, there are no risks of side effects.

It is important to note that there are three different types of olive oil:

- Refined olive oil
- Virgin olive oil
- Extra Virgin olive oil

Extra virgin olive oil is the least processed variety and is considered to be the healthiest of the three. The oil is extracted using natural methods and standardized for purity and certain sensory qualities, such as taste and smell.

In addition, extra virgin olive oil has the most antioxidants of all three of the olive oils. Use it in place of other oils and you will be reaping the benefits of this wonderful heart-healthy monounsaturated fat!

Spice Things Up

Instead of reaching for the salt shaker, why not use fresh or dried spices. We will cover herbs and spices more in depth later in the book but just know that most of them come with powerful antioxidants.

Reduce processed sugars and sweet treats. They are known for triggering the release of cytokines which are inflammatory messengers

It is important to read your labels because sugar has a sneaky unnecessary way of being included in manufactured foods. For example, yogurt, ketchup, salad dressing, and pasta sauce just to name a few. Watch for words like high fructose corn syrup and sucrose - stay away from those.

Your sugar intake should be less than 10% of your daily caloric intake. Today there are so many healthy options, you can always find a healthy product to substitute a product high in sugar. Yogurt for example, in my opinion tastes so much better without the high fructose corn syrup - so much better. You will probably notice the difference right away - in a good way!

Go Fish

While trans and saturated fats have a bad reputation, cold water fish, including salmon, anchovy, tuna, herring, sardines, and halibut, are all rich in inflammation-fighting omega-3 fatty acids.

Omega-3s are a type of a polyunsaturated fat known for its powerful anti-inflammatory properties, particularly by reducing two inflammatory proteins.

Try to eat at least three to four ounces of fish per week. It's so good for you!

Cut Out Trans Fats Altogether

Trans fat was made with good intentions as a healthier alternative to butter, but we now know better. Strong evidence discourages its use due to its inflammatory and negative effects on human health. It is bad, bad, bad.

Trans fats are commonly found in margarines, fried foods, prepackaged snacks, and desserts. Watch out for words like" hydrogenated oils" and "hydrogenated" products - this is trans fats. Instead of margarine, choose real butter.

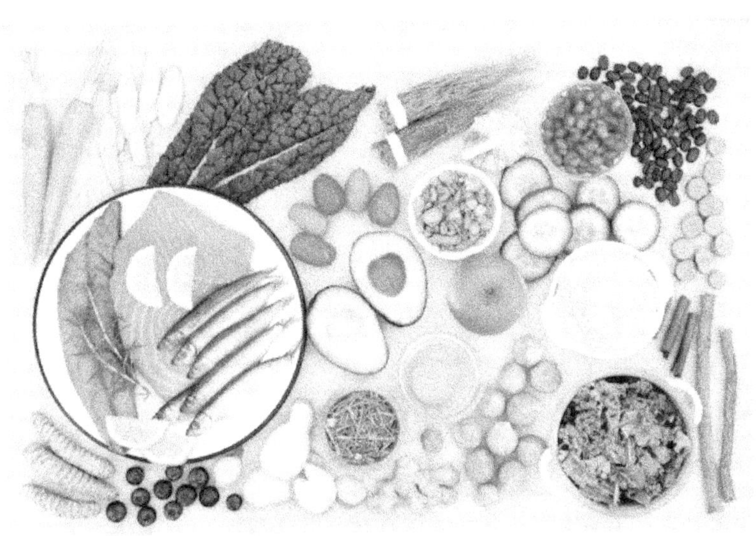

Anti-Inflammatory Foods

The best things about the anti-inflammatory diet are that it isn't too restrictive and it's delicious. There's so much to choose from, it literally is what you make of it. Variety is the key.

It is comprised of fresh colorful fruits and vegetables, fiber-rich whole grains, healthy fats, fresh herbs, and spices. It is pretty safe to say that if you like the Mediterranean Diet, you will probably enjoy this diet too. Both diets focus on healthy fats and nutrient-dense foods like nuts, salmon, olive oil, and avocado.

Some of the compounds and nutrients that you will hear about over and over again with this diet are resveratrol, turmeric, anthocyanins, and omega-3 fatty acids.

Resveratrol is an antioxidant found in grapes, red wine, white wine grape juice, peanuts, cocoa, blueberries, bilberries, and cranberries.

Turmeric is best known in the U.S. as a spice but in other parts of the world, it is used to treat many health conditions. It is believed to have anti-inflammatory, antioxidant, and perhaps even anticancer properties. There are several ways to use turmeric in your meals. A few are listed below.

- Add it to your eggs - If you don't eat eggs, you can add it to a tofu scramble, for example.
- Sprinkle it on veggies
- Make Golden Milk (see the recipe on page 64) - Relax with a soothing cup in the evening.
- Add it to Smoothies
- Add a dash to your soups

Anthocyanins are antioxidants found in red, blue, and purple fruits and vegetables. They belong to the same flavonoid family as the antioxidants found in dark chocolate, tea, and wine. Foods containing anthocyanins have been used for years as natural remedies. These antioxidants are believed to help prevent and treat conditions associated with inflammation. The foods below contain the highest amount of anthocyanins:

- Mulberries
- Black chokeberries
- Black elderberries
- Black currants
- Sweet cherries
- Blackberries
- Lingonberries
- Strawberries
- Sour cherries
- Red raspberries
- Black grapes
- Plums
- Blueberries
- Black beans
- Red currants
- Red wine
- Red onions

There are many different sources of omega-3 fatty acids. The foods listed below have some of the highest amounts:

- Mackerel
- Salmon
- Cod Liver Oil
- Herring
- Oysters
- Sardines
- Anchovies
- Caviar
- Flaxseed
- Chia Seeds
- Walnuts
- Soybeans

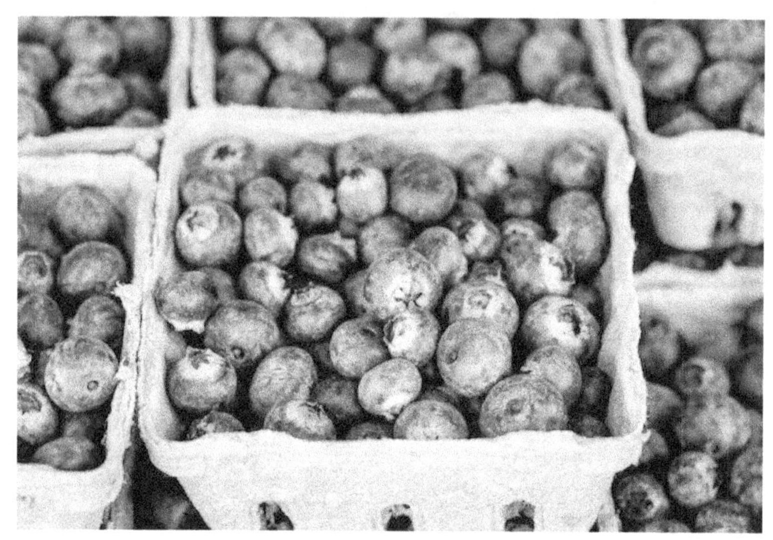

Most Powerful Foods

Avocados

Avocados come with a long list of health benefits, but it is the sugars found in avocados that may make them particularly good at reducing inflammation.

Studies have found avocados to be effective in blocking the inflammatory response in specific cells involved in the body's immune response. One study in particular involved participants where one group ate burgers with a slice of avocado and another set of participants ate the burger without avocado. Those who ate the burger with the added avocado had much lower levels of inflammatory markers following the meal. This is just one example.

Beans

Beans are so good for you! They are high in fiber and phytonutrients which reduce inflammation. They are also high in protein and have a low score on the glycemic index. Try to eat one cup of beans at least twice a week. More often would be even better.

Berries

Naturally high in antioxidants, berries are one of the most healthy foods. Blueberries are especially powerful because they contain quercetin, which has strong-anti-inflammatory properties.

Broccoli

Broccoli absolutely deserves the title of anti-inflammatory super powerful food. In addition to being associated with decreased risk of heart disease and certain cancers, it is also one of the best natural sources of sulforaphane which is a powerful antioxidant with anti-inflammatory properties.

Celery

Celery is a very powerful anti-inflammatory. It is rich in flavonoids which have been found to lower inflammation, improve blood pressure, and cholesterol levels.

Cherries

Packed full of antioxidants like catechins and anthocyanins, cherries are very effective at decreasing oxidative stress and fighting inflammation. Both sweet and tart cherries have been shown to contain antioxidants that reduce inflammation.

Chili peppers and bell peppers

Bell peppers (especially the red ones) contain loads of vitamin C and inflammation- fighting antioxidants, like beta-carotene, quercetin, and luteolin. Chili peppers contain sinapic acid and ferulic acid, both of which work to reduce inflammation and oxidative stress in the body. Both mild and spicy varieties of peppers have super beneficial anti-inflammatory qualities.

Dark Chocolate

Dark chocolate that has 70 percent or more cocoa is highly rich in antioxidants which have anti-inflammatory effects. The flavanols in dark chocolate help to reduce inflammation and keep the cells that line the arteries healthy.

Get your chocolate fix with a square of dark chocolate. Just remember that it needs to be at least 70 percent cacao to reap the anti-inflammatory benefits.

Ginger

Ginger contains several active compounds, including gingerol, that give it its anti-inflammatory power. You can drink ginger tea, add it to stir-fry, or in ginger based salad dressings, etc.

Grapes

All grapes, red, purple, and green are packed with antioxidants. They contain anthocyanins and resveratrol, both of which have been shown to reduce inflammation. Tip: You can freeze grapes. I love to add them to my glasses of water and smoothies.

Green Tea

All tea is considered anti-inflammatory because it contains antioxidants called catechins, which reduce inflammation. But Green Tea has the most benefits because it contains EGCG, the most powerful type of catechin.

Leafy Greens

Spinach, kale, collard greens and other leafy greens are packed with antioxidants. Spinach, in particular, is rich in vitamin A, an antioxidant that helps fight cell damage that can lead to age-related vision problems like macular degeneration.

Mushrooms

Mushrooms are rich in selenium, B vitamins, copper, phenols, and other antioxidants that provide anti-inflammatory protection against inflammatory conditions such as inflammatory bowel disease. Studies have shown that overcooking mushrooms can reduce the power of its anti-inflammatory compounds drastically. To reap the anti-inflammatory benefits of mushrooms, eat them lightly cooked or raw.

Pineapple

Pineapple is the only dietary source of the anti-inflammatory compound bromelain. Bromelain is a protein-digesting enzyme known for its anti-inflammatory properties. In addition, pineapple is a great source of fiber, potassium, and vitamin C.

Salmon

Salmon is an excellent source of protein and omega-3 fatty acids.
The omega 3's in salmon have been shown to have strong anti-inflammatory properties. To reap the benefits, try to have salmon at least once a week.

Tomatoes and tomato juice are both packed full of several antioxidants with powerful anti-inflammatory properties, such as vitamin C, lycopene, and potassium. Tomatoes happen to be the richest source of lycopene in the traditional western diet. Lycopene is particularly effective at reducing inflammation, as well as the risk of certain cancers and heart disease. Cooking tomatoes in olive oil can increase your ability to absorb lycopene when you eat them, as the cooking process appears to make the lycopene more available.

Turmeric

Turmeric, a spice derived from the rhizome of the Curcuma longa plant, has long been recognized for its medicinal properties. The beneficial effects of turmeric include anti-inflammatory, antimicrobial, and antioxidant activity.

Turmeric is composed of approximately two to five percent curcumin, its most active component, commonly found in supplement form. However, research has found that several of the health benefits of this spice occur independently of curcumin, which suggests there may be additional benefits to consuming whole turmeric.

Walnuts

Walmunts stand out from the rest of the nuts because they are the highest in ALA, an omega-3 fatty acid that has potent anti-inflammatory effects. Walnuts are also a rich source of anti-inflammatory vitamins and antioxidants, including vitamin E and other phytonutrients like phenolic acids and flavonoids.
Research suggests that it only takes about 7 walnuts per day to benefit from them.

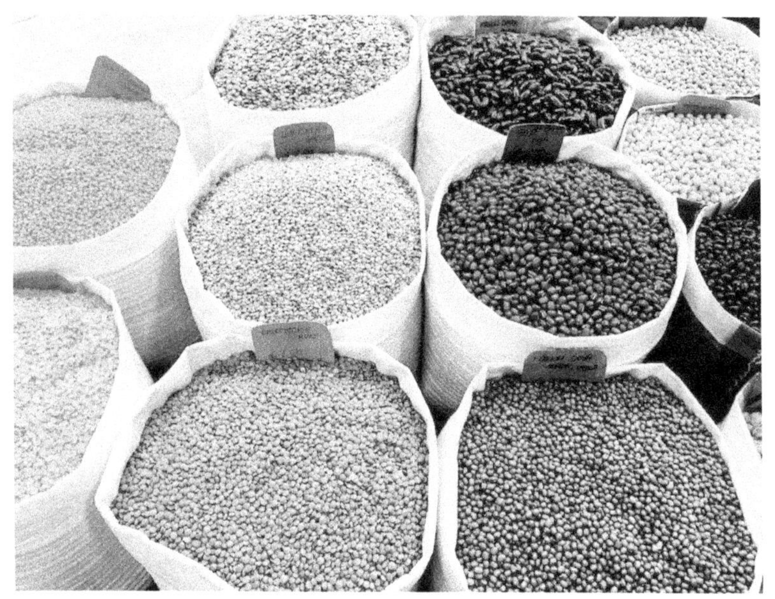

Anti-Inflammatory Food List

Now that we have covered the most powerful anti-inflammatory foods, let's take a look at the rest. If you are not already consuming some of the foods below, try to start incorporating them into your diet in place of foods that either cause inflammation or don't have anti-inflammatory properties.

Anti-Inflammatory Vegetables

Artichoke

The flavonoid rutin which is known for its antioxidant and anti-inflammatory properties is found in the leaves of artichoke.

Arugula

Arugula contains isothiocyanates and 3-carbinol which studies have shown to suppress inflammation in the body. These bioactive compounds control oxidative stress and reduce inflammation.

Asparagus

Asparagus contains many saponins, flavonoids, and other phenolics with strong antioxidant and anti-inflammatory effects. .

Bamboo Shoots

Bamboo Shoots contain phenolic acids which have antimicrobial and anti-inflammatory qualities. They are a great source of vitamins and minerals including vitamin C, manganese, and magnesium.

Beans

Beans, like several of the foods that you will see on this list have already been mentioned in the previous section. But, beans are so good for you they are worth mentioning again, and again. They are high in fiber and phytonutrients which reduce inflammation. They are also high in protein and have a low score on the glycemic index.

Beets

Beets contain betalains which give them their vibrant red color. Their high concentration of betalains possess anti-inflammatory properties which can reduce inflammation throughout the entire body.

Bok Choy

Bok Choy contains selenium which prevents inflammation.

Broccoli

As mentioned in the previous section, broccoli is rich in sulforaphane, an antioxidant that decreases inflammation by reducing your levels of cytokines and nuclear factor kappa B which are molecules that drive inflammation in your body.

Brussel Sprouts

Brussels sprouts help regulate inflammation because they are packed with alpha-lipoic acid which is an antioxidant that is exceptionally good at reducing inflammation.

Cabbage

Cabbage contains glutamine, an amino acid that is a strong anti-inflammatory agent. Cabbage is actually considered one of the top food sources of glutamine.

Carrots

Carrots contain carotenoids which have antioxidant and anti-inflammatory properties.

Cauliflower

Cauliflower contains the compound sulforaphane which reduces the inflammatory damage caused by oxidative stress.

Celery

As mentioned in the previous section, celery is a strong anti-inflammatory, rich in flavonoids which have been found to lower inflammation, improve blood pressure, and cholesterol levels.

Chard

Chard is loaded with vitamins A, K, and C, giving it plenty of health benefits. When it comes to inflammation, its vitamin A and K content is what makes it helpful. Both of these vitamins help reduce inflammation in different ways. Vitamin A boosts our immune system and vitamin K supports bone and blood health keeping inflammation in check.

Cucumber

Cucumbers are great for inflammation because they contain polyphenols. They can reduce inflammation externally too when applied directly to the skin.

Eggplant

Eggplant contains chlorogenic acid, an antioxidant that helps fight free radical damage and inflammation.

Garlic

Garlic limits the effects of pro-inflammatory cytokines.

Hearts of Palm

Hearts of palm are rich in polyphenols which work to neutralize free-radical damage in the body. Polyphenols also have strong anti-inflammatory benefits and prebiotics, meaning they feed the beneficial bacteria in your gut.

Kale

One cup of kale contains 10 percent of the recommended daily amount of omega-3 fatty acids, which reduces inflammation in the body. Kale's sulfur-containing phytochemicals can also aid in the maintenance of the body's natural inflammatory response.

Leeks

Leeks are rich in flavonoids which are antioxidants that have anti-inflammatory properties.

Mushrooms

Mushrooms contain healthy compounds called beta-glucans, which have anti-inflammatory properties.

Onion

Onions contain an antioxidant called

quercetin. Quercetin is an anti-inflammatory.

Peppers

Bell peppers (especially the red ones) contain loads of vitamin C and inflammation fighting antioxidants, like beta-carotene, quercetin, and luteolin. Chili peppers contain sinapic acid and ferulic acid, both of which work to reduce inflammation and oxidative stress in the body.

Rhubarb

Rhubarb is rich in antioxidants, particularly anthocyanins and proanthocyanidins. These antioxidants have antibacterial, anti-inflammatory, and anti-cancer properties.

Spinach

Spinach is full of quercetin, a powerful antioxidant that has anti-inflammatory properties.

String Beans

Green beans or string beans contain carotenoids and are an excellent source of vitamin A. One cup of green beans offers close to 20 percent of the daily value for vitamin A. This nutrient fights inflammation and boosts immunity.

Tomatoes

Tomatoes contain the healthy nutrients and compounds lycopene, beta carotene, and vitamin C all of which act as antioxidants and exert anti-inflammatory effects in the body.

Water Chestnuts

Water chestnuts contain the antioxidants fisetin, diosmetin, luteolin, and tectorigenin, which can help repair damaged cells and reduce inflammation.

Yellow Squash

The anti-inflammatory activity of squash

is due to the presence of omega-3 fatty acids, carotenoids like lutein, zeaxanthin, and beta-carotene.

Zucchini

The beta-carotene and vitamin C found in zucchini both have anti-inflammatory properties.

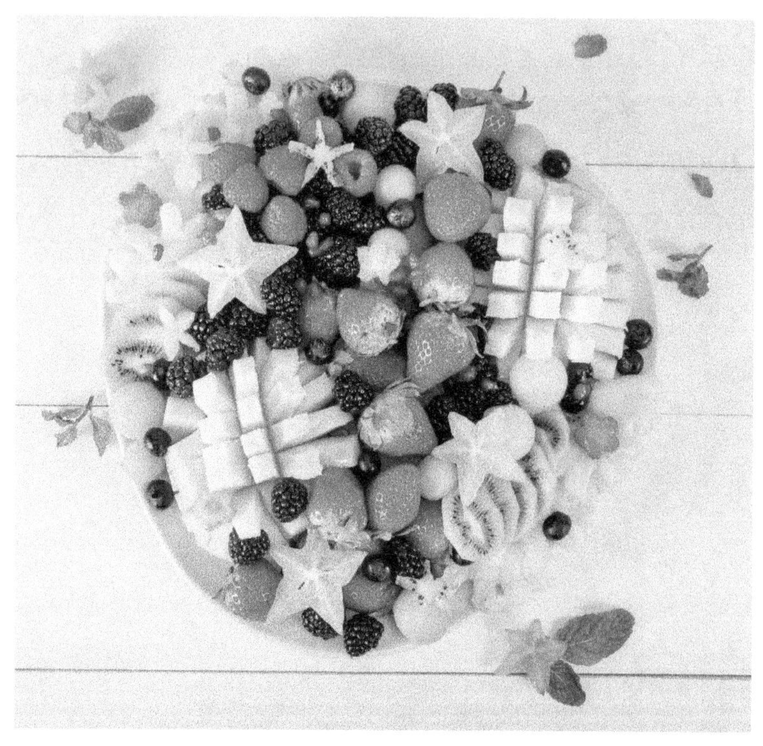

Anti-Inflammatory Fruits

Apples

Apples are rich in polyphenols that reduce inflammation.

Apricots

Apricots are a strong dietary source of catechins. These phytonutrients are potent anti-inflammatory nutrients.

Bananas

Bananas are high in prebiotics that stimulate the immune system through their effect on the gut microbiota. They also reduce inflammation by increasing anti-inflammatory cytokines while decreasing pro-inflammatory cytokines.

Berries

As discussed previously, berries are among the healthiest foods. Blueberries are especially powerful because they contain quercetin, which has strong-anti-inflammatory properties.

Cantaloupe

Cantaloupe contains antioxidants that help prevent oxidative stress and anti-inflammatory phytonutrients including the carotenoids alpha-carotene, beta-carotene, and lutein.

Cherries

As discussed previously, cherries are loaded with antioxidants like catechins and anthocyanins, which are very effective at decreasing oxidative stress and fighting inflammation. Both sweet and tart cherries have been shown to contain antioxidants that reduce inflammation.

Clementine

Clementines are rich in flavonoids that can help reduce inflammation.

Figs

Figs are loaded with antioxidants that stop free radicals from damaging cells and creating new inflammation in the body. They are also packed with phytochemicals that help with reducing inflammation.

Grapes

Grapes contain various phytonutrients. Among those phytonutrients in grapes, the most well known is resveratrol, an antioxidant found in the skin of grapes that has anti-inflammatory properties.

Kiwi

Kiwi contain vitamin C and vitamin E, and are an excellent source of plant compounds that have antioxidant and anti-inflammatory effects in the body.

Lemon

Lemons are rich in flavonoid have anti-inflammatory properties.

Mango

Mangos contain mangiferin which has

antioxidant and anti-inflammatory properties.

Olives

There are two antioxidants found in olives, hydroxytyrosol and oleanolic acid that have been effective in reducing inflammation.

Oranges

Oranges contain flavonoids. Studies indicate that citrus flavonoids protect the cells against the damage of free radicals, can reduce inflammation, and provide therapeutic benefits.

Papaya

Papaya is loaded with antioxidants that can reduce inflammation, fight disease and help keep you looking young. They have impressive levels of vitamins A, C, and E. They also contain the enzyme papain, which is known to lessen inflammation and are very high in carotenoids that can help to reduce inflammation.

Pear

Pears, especially those with colorful skins, provide phytonutrients known to help keep inflammation low by neutralizing free radicals.

Pineapple

As discussed previously, pineapple is the only dietary source of the anti-inflammatory compound bromelain. Bromelain is a protein-digesting enzyme known for its anti-inflammatory properties. In addition, pineapple is a great source of fiber, potassium, and vitamin C.

Plums

Plums are great sources of vitamins C and E. They also contain anthocyanins which are known for their anti-inflammatory properties.

Pomegranate

Pomegranates contain ellagitannins that have anti-inflammatory effects on the cells in the body. Ellagitannins are bioactive polyphenols, chemical compounds found in the peel and seeds of pomegranate.

StarFruit

The high levels of antioxidants in star fruit make it a great anti-inflammatory. It is also high in fiber and can help boost your metabolism which makes it great for weight loss too.

Strawberries

As discussed in the previous section, all berries have anti-inflammatory benefits. Strawberries, blackberries, blueberries, and cranberries are particularly potent in antioxidant and anti-inflammatory activity.

Watermelon

Watermelon contains antioxidants, lycopene, and vitamin C which can lower inflammation and oxidative stress.

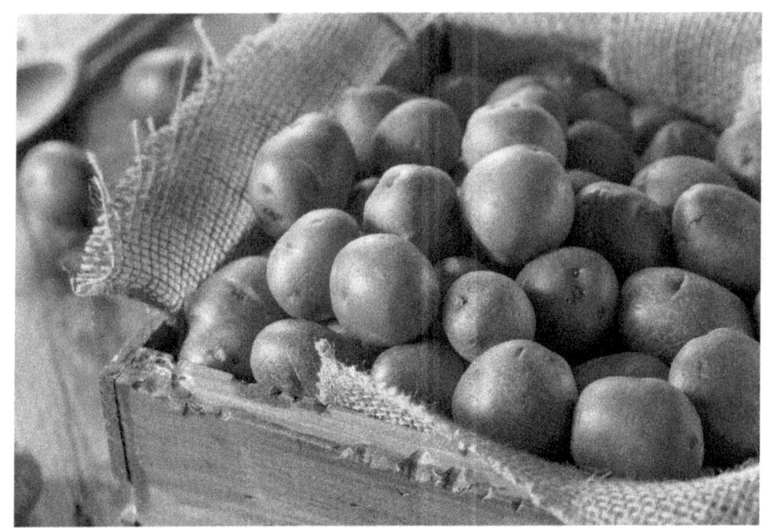

Anti-Inflammatory Starchy Vegetables

The starchy vegetables listed below are high in fiber, naturally gluten free and are also high in essential vitamins and minerals. They are excellent additions to an anti-inflammatory diet, and are great carb replacements for breads and pastas.

Parsnips

Parsnips have anti-inflammatory properties due to the active plant compounds furanocoumarins, flavonoids, and polyacetylenes.

Potatoes

Yellow and purple potatoes are high in antioxidants such as phenols, carotenoids, and anthocyanins. Research suggests these antioxidants may help fight inflammation and reduce the risk of inflammation-related conditions.

Pumpkin

Pumpkin is full of anti-inflammatory influencers like beta-carotene, alpha-carotene, and lutein. These antioxidants help protect your immune cells and fight off free radicals.

Red Potatoes

Red potatoes contain phenolic

compounds. These compounds help to neutralize harmful free radicals in the body and decrease inflammation.

Spaghetti Squash

Spaghetti squash contains omega 3 and omega 6 essential fatty acids. These essential fatty acids are known to have anti-inflammatory effects.

Sweet Potatoes

Sweet Potatoes are a great source of choline and anthocyanins which have powerful anti-inflammatory properties.

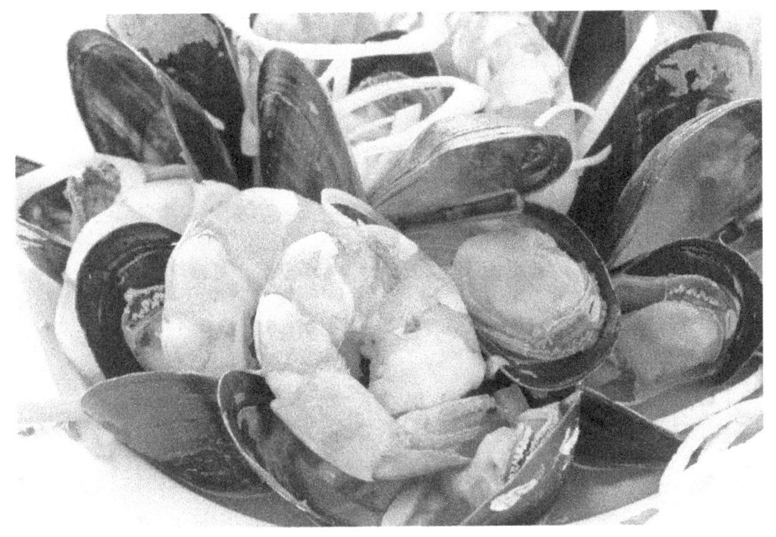

Anti-Inflammatory Proteins

Fatty fish like salmon, tuna, mackerel and sardines are some of the best choices in the anti-inflammatory protein category. Other protein choices include omega-3 enriched eggs, natural cheeses, yogurt, and lean meats, like skinless poultry. Plus, there are also some vegetarian/vegan options listed below.

Bluefin Tuna

Rich in omega-3, vitamin B12 and several other vitamins and minerals, the health benefits of Bluefin Tuna are quite impressive.

Bluefin Tuna can also keep the body's overall stress levels down by reducing inflammation because of the anti-inflammatory agents in omega-3.

Clams

Clams are loaded with nutrients and are especially high in iron and vitamin B12. They are also a great source of omega-3 fatty acids which as previously discussed, have anti-inflammatory properties.

Crab

Crab is a good source of omega 3 fatty acids which have anti-inflammatory properties. It also contains astaxanthin which has been shown to have powerful anti-inflammatory effects.

Crawfish

Crawfish are a good source of protein, vitamins, and minerals. They are low in calories and fat, and they contain omega 3 fatty acids. Crawfish are also a good source of antioxidants and have anti-inflammatory properties.

Flounder

Founder is high in fatty acids like Omega 3, which have anti-inflammatory properties. These properties are beneficial not only for treating inflammation but also for preventing other diseases associated with inflammation.

Halibut

Halibut contains the nutrients niacin, selenium, and omega-3 fatty acids, which all have anti-inflammatory properties.

Herring

Herring is very high In omega 3 fatty acids.

Lobster

The protein and healthy fat composition of lobster can help reduce inflammation in the body. The omega 3 fatty acids in shellfish regulate cholesterol levels and enhance the molecules that defend the body, known as prostaglandins.

MahiMahi

Mahi mahi contains omega 3 fatty acids.

Mackerel

Mackerel is rich in omega 3 and omega-6 fatty acids, as well as vitamin A, B6, B12, C, D, E, K,   a wide range of important minerals, and protein.

Mussels

Mussels are rich in zinc and omega-3 fatty

acids, both have anti-inflammatory properties and help to reduce inflammation.

Oysters

Oysters are abundant in omega-3 fatty acids.

Salmon

As discussed previously, Salmon is an excellent source of protein and has a long chain of omega 3 fatty acids that have been shown to have strong anti-inflammatory properties after your body metabolizes the acids into compounds called protectins and resolvins. To reap the anti-inflammatory benefits of salmon, try to have it once a week.

Sardines

Sardines are loaded with important nutrients like Omega 3 fatty acids, iodine and Vitamin D. In fact, one sardine contains approximately 60 percent of an individual's recommended daily intake of omega 3 fatty acids. Both fresh and canned sardines have health benefits. These include fighting inflammation and supporting the health of your heart, bones, and immune system.

Shrimp

Shrimp are rich in nutrients including a wide variety of vitamins, minerals, proteins, and omega-3 fatty acids.

Snapper

Snapper is rich in selenium, vitamin A, potassium, and omega 3 fatty acids. As we know, omega 3 fatty acids are important for countering inflammation, lowering your risk of heart disease, and lowering triglycerides.

Striped Bass

Striped Bass offers a significant amount of protein, omega-3 fatty acids, essential amino acids, and select vitamins and minerals.

Tempeh

Tempeh is a product similar to tofu in that it is made from soybeans and is frequently eaten by vegetarians as a meat substitute. Tempeh differs from tofu in that tempeh is created through a process of fermentation, whereas tofu is not. Because of the fermentation, tempeh has a number of different health benefits. Tempeh has protein content comparable to that of meat and contains many important vitamins and minerals. It has a relatively firm texture and, like tofu, tends to take on the flavor of whatever it is cooked with. The isoflavones found in tempeh are known to be an effective anti-inflammatory.

Trout

Trout is a great source of omega 3s.

Tofu

Tofu contains several anti-inflammatory and antioxidant phyto-chemicals making it a great addition to an anti-inflammatory diet. Tofu is also a good source of protein because it has a well-balanced amino acid profile. It is also a good source of fiber, potassium, magnesium, iron, copper, and manganese.

Tuna

Tuna is a great source of omega 3 fatty acids and vitamin D. As we know, omega 3s are known for their anti-inflammatory properties. Tuna also contains vitamins B-12, selenium, and zinc.

Does it matter if you have canned versus fresh tuna? The truth is there isn't a huge nutritional difference between canned and fresh tuna. Although fresh tuna will have a slightly higher protein content along with no carbohydrates, canned tuna actually features mostly the same amount of vitamins and nutrients. Most canned tuna are made from cheaper tuna such as skipjack or albacore tuna. It also depends on whether it's packed in oil or water.

If you like the convenience of canned tuna, you can get higher-quality versions of canned tuna. It usually comes in jars with larger pieces of the fish and is preserved in olive oil. The higher quality tuna is more expensive but the flavor and texture make it worth it.

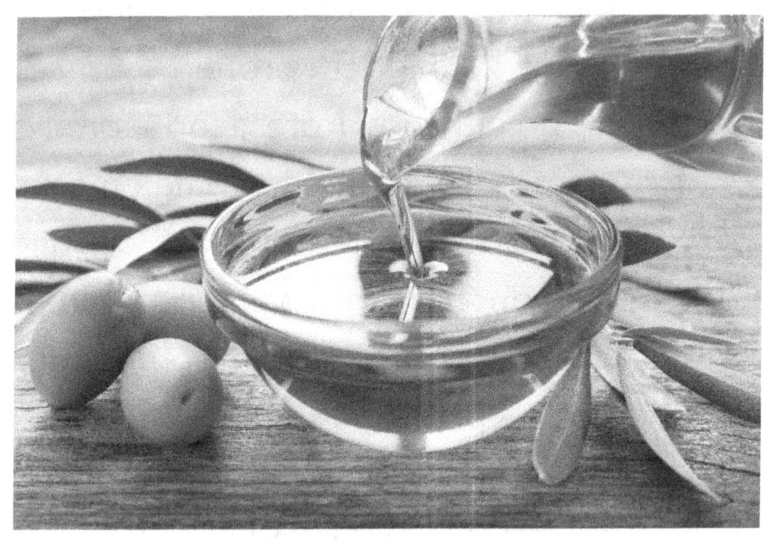

Anti-Inflammatory Fats & Oils

Almond Oil

Almond oil is full of monounsaturated fatty acids. It has high levels of antioxidants which gives it the ability to decrease inflammation.

When cooking with almond oil, remember to keep the heat at a low temperature to prevent burning the oil and destroying the nutritional value. It is best used for salad dressing, or low-heat baking.

Avocado Oil

Similar to olive oil, avocado oil is high in unsaturated fats which are linked to lowering inflammation.

Kitchen tip: Avocado oil has a mild flavor and a higher smoke point than most plant oils, so it performs well for high-heat cooking such as stir-frying.

Hemp Seed Oil

The gamma-linoleic acid found in hemp seed oil has been shown to reduce inflammation.

Extra Virgin Olive Oil

As discussed previously, extra virgin olive oil can reduce inflammation. Its main anti-inflammatory effects are from the antioxidant oleocanthal. In addition, the antioxidants in olive oil can reduce oxidative damage due to free radicals. Research has also shown that oleic acid, which is the main fatty acid in olive oil, can reduce levels of inflammatory markers.

Flaxseed Oil

Flaxseed oil is high in omega-3's.

Almonds

Compared to other nuts, almonds have a higher amount of fiber with three grams per ounce. Consuming enough fiber during the day not only helps with reducing inflammation it can also assist with weight management and lowers cholesterol.

Almonds are known for being a rich source of vitamin E, and research shows that a diet rich in almonds can help with lowering markers of inflammation.

Avocado

Avocados are a great source of healthy monounsaturated fat and antioxidants, which can lessen your body's inflammatory response. In fact, the anti-inflammatory properties of avocados are so strong that they may actually offset less healthy food choices.

Brazil Nuts

Brazil nuts have several antioxidants, including vitamin E and phenols. Antioxidants can help to fight free radicals, reducing oxidative stress and inflammation in your body.

Chia Seeds

Caffeic acid, an antioxidant found in chia seeds, can help to fight inflammation in the body. Eating chia seeds regularly may also help to reduce inflammatory markers, which often indicate the presence of an inflammatory disease.

Flax Seeds

Two tablespoons of ground flaxseed contain over 140 percent of the daily value of omega 3 fatty acids, which are known to fight inflammation. The alpha-linolenic acid in the seeds was found to decrease pro-inflammatory compounds in the body.

Hazel Nuts

Hazel Nuts are considered to be the second richest source of monounsaturated fatty acids and are known to be an excellent anti-inflammatory food. Hazelnuts are also a hypolipidemic food, meaning it is lower in saturated fat and a good heart-healthy choice due to their ability to lower LDL cholesterol levels - commonly linked to increased inflammation and chronic disease risk.

Hemp Seeds

The amount of omega-3s in hemp seeds and the seeds healthful omega-3s to omega-6 ratio can together help to reduce inflammation. In addition, hemp seeds are a rich source of gamma linolenic acid, a polyunsaturated fatty acid which may also have anti-inflammatory effects.

Macadamia Nuts

Macadamia nuts have some of the highest flavonoid levels of all tree nuts. This antioxidant fights inflammation and helps lower cholesterol.

Olives

Olives are rich in anti-inflammatory and antioxidant properties. 3.5 ounces of olives contains 10.9 grams of fat, 74 percent from oleic acid associated with decreased inflammation. They are also packed with antioxidant polyphenol compounds.

Pecans

Pecans are rich in omega-3 fatty acids, which is key to decreasing inflammation in the body. They can also reduce inflammation by reducing the formation of inflammatory mediator molecules. And, they can help counteract any pro-inflammatory activity happening from overconsuming saturated fatty acids.

Pistachios

Pistachios are rich in multiple antioxidants and are known for reducing oxidative stress that can lead to increased LDL cholesterol.

Oxidative stress causes an imbalance of reactive oxygen species, which can lead to chronic inflammation. Diets rich in polyphenols, like the kind found in pistachios, are key for reducing oxidative stress and inflammatory activity.

Pumpkin Seeds

Pumpkin seeds contain antioxidants including phenols and flavonoids. Phenols help fend off cell-damaging compounds in the body, which may protect against aging and disease. Flavonoids counter compounds that damage healthy cells and have strong anti-inflammatory effects.

Sesame Seeds

Sesame seeds are rich in antioxidants and anti-inflammatory compounds such as sesamin, Sesamolinol, and vitamin E. Their nutrients help to protect cells from damage and reduce inflammation throughout the body.

Sunflower seeds contain vitamin E, flavonoids, and other plant compounds that can reduce inflammation. A study found that consuming sunflower seeds five or more times each week resulted in lower levels of inflammation.

As mentioned previously, out of every nut to choose from, walnuts are one of the best for reducing inflammation due to their high concentration of alpha-linolenic acid which is a type of omega-3 fatty acid.

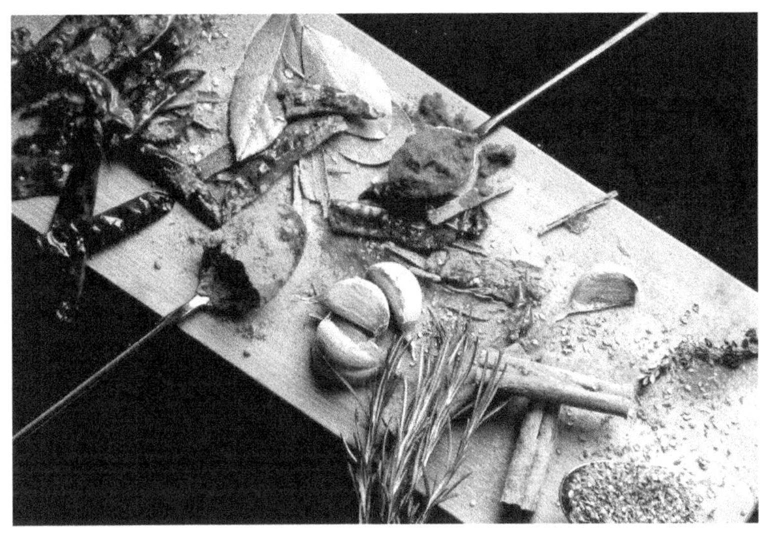

Anti-Inflammatory Herbs & Spices

Basil

Basil contains powerful essential oils, including eugenol, citronellol, and linalool. Findings from many studies have indicated that these enzyme-inhibiting oils help lower inflammation.

Black Pepper

Black pepper has both anti-inflammatory and pain-reducing properties. Piperine, a compound that gives black pepper its sharp taste, prevents and reduces inflammation.

Cayenne Pepper

Cayenne peppers have been praised for their health benefits since ancient times. They contain a compound called capsaicinoids. This is what gives it its anti-inflammatory properties.

Cilantro

Studies have found a range of antimicrobial, antioxidant, and anti-inflammatory health benefits. In addition, it has been shown to protect against cellular damage, help treat infections, and guard against oxidative stress by absorbing and neutralizing free radicals.

Cinnamon

Researchers have identified many different types of flavonoids in cinnamon, all of which are highly effective in fighting inflammation levels throughout the body.

Clove

Cloves contain eugenol, a photogenic bioactive component that has antioxidant and anti-inflammatory properties.

Curry

Curry contains spices like turmeric, coriander, and chili pepper so it is no wonder that the seasoning has been shown to provide anti-inflammatory benefits.

Dill

Dill contains flavonoids which have potent antioxidant and anti-inflammatory properties.

Ginger

Ginger has served as a holistic medicine for centuries. The compound that is most responsible for ginger's medicinal properties is gingerol. As the main bioactive compound, research indicates that gingerol may reduce oxidative stress, which is associated with inflammation.

Garlic

Garlic contains diallyl disulfide, an anti-inflammatory compound that limits the effects of pro-inflammatory cytokines.

Mint

Mint plants contain an antioxidant and

anti-inflammatory agent called rosmarinic acid.

Oregano

Studies have shown that in addition to being an antimicrobial, oregano is also a potent anti-inflammatory due to the compounds carvacrol and thymol that are present in it.

Parsley

Parsley contains eugenol which has anti-inflammatory properties.

Rosemary

Rosemary offers antioxidant and anti-inflammatory benefits due to its polyphenolic compounds of rosmarinic acid and carnosic acid.

Sage

Sage contains carnosic acid and carnosol. These both have antioxidant and anti-inflammatory properties.

Thyme

Thyme contains the compound thymol. Research suggests that thymol has anti-inflammatory properties.

Turmeric

We have already discussed the benefits of turmeric but because it fits into the herb and spice category, I wanted to include it here again for quick reference. We know that turmeric is a spice derived from the rhizome of the Curcuma longa plant, and has long been recognized for its medicinal properties. The beneficial effects of turmeric include anti-inflammatory, antimicrobial, and antioxidant activity. Turmeric is composed of approximately two to five percent curcumin, its most active component, commonly found in supplement form.

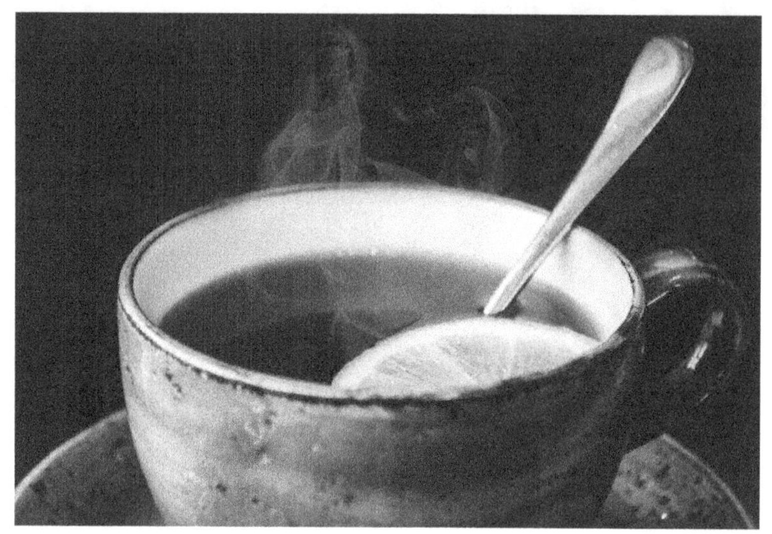

Tea Time

Green Tea

You have probably heard that green tea is one of the healthiest beverages you can drink. Many of its benefits are due to its antioxidant and anti-inflammatory properties, especially a substance called EGCG which inhibits inflammation by reducing pro-inflammatory cytokine production and damage to the fatty acids in your cells.

Matcha

Matcha is a type of green tea that has been used for centuries in China and Japan. The leaves are harvested, steamed, dried, and then ground into a fine powder. When that powder is added to hot water and blended with a whisk, it creates a sweet, creamy flavor and texture different from other teas. It can be enjoyed hot or iced.

Matcha contains high amounts of substances with antioxidant and anti-inflammatory effects. The antioxidants in matcha protect cells from the effects of free-radicals and support your immune system. This can help lower inflammation in the body.

Black Tea

The anti-inflammatory power of black tea stems from the two flavonoids it contains - thearubigins and theaflavin. These two compounds inhibit inflammatory enzymes which can control and eliminate free radicals within the body.

While black tea is the most processed of the three teas, it carries many of the same research-proven benefits as green tea. The way that tea acts in our bodies is very individualized, for some tea drinkers, it may have too much caffeine.

Research shows that black tea has properties that provide protection against inflammation and inflammatory conditions.

White

White teas have excellent anti-inflammatory properties. The EGCG found in it is known to fight atherosclerosis which is caused by inflammation due to environmental pollutants. It is also good for the flu and colds because it kills various bacteria and viruses including the virus that causes influenza.

Ginger

Ginger tea is made from its root. It is then sliced, dried and ground into a powder. The compounds contained in ginger are gingerol and shogaol which fight inflammation and oxidative stress. Ginger is a very effective remedy for inflammation as well as the pain associated with inflammation. It also works really well as a remedy for nausea - it works!

Rooibos

Rooibos tea is native to South Africa but is easily available for anyone thanks to the internet and can be found in most health food stores. It contains polyphenols and has the ability to act as a natural antioxidant and anti-inflammatory. And, it is delicious!

Turmeric Tea

Turmeric is a powerful anti-inflammatory root that has been used for many years as a medicinal tea. It contains curcumin, known to fight inflammation and is in the same family as ginger. There are many types of turmeric tea. My favorite is a Ginger Peach Turmeric combo - I love it! You can find the packaged tea bags at most grocery and health food stores but I have also included some recipes below to make your own turmeric tea at home. There is also a recipe for Golden Milk in the Breakfast section.

Spicy Turmeric Tea

This tea is immune-boosting and full of flavor. It is the perfect tea for colds, has lots of anti-inflammatory properties, and is so easy to make.

Anti-Inflammatory Ingredients: turmeric, ginger, cinnamon, lemon juice

Servings: 5
Time: 15 minutes

Ingredients

2 tsp ground turmeric
2 tsp ground ginger
1 cinnamon stick
1-2 tbsp raw honey
5-7 cups water
1 tsp lemon juice

In a medium size pot, add all ingredients, stir, bring to a boil and stir again. Let the tea simmer for about 15 minutes, strain, serve, and enjoy the goodness!

Homemade Chai Tea

This recipe is inspired by traditional versions from India. It makes a savory aromatic blend of anti-inflammatory ingredients.

Anti-Inflammatory Ingredients: black tea, cinnamon, cloves, ginger

Servings: 2
Time: 15 minutes

Ingredients

3 cups of almond milk

3 black tea bags

1 tsp ground cinnamon

½ tsp ground ginger

¼ tsp ground cloves

⅛ tsp ground cardamom

½ tsp vanilla extract

2 tbsp raw honey

Heat the almond milk in a small pot over medium heat. When it starts to simmer, turn off heat and add tea bags. Let the tea steep for 5 minutes and then remove the tea bags.

Turn the heat to medium, add cinnamon, ginger, clever, cardamom, vanilla, and honey. Whisk until the tea is hot, careful not to boil.

Pour the tea in a tea or coffee cup and sprinkle with cinnamon. Enjoy!

Note: Because this recipe uses ground spices, you will have some sediment at the bottom of your cup. To prevent this, just strain the tea as you pour it into your cup.

Lemon Ginger Ice Tea

This recipe makes a one gallon pitcher of tea. To make less, you can cut the recipe in half.

Anti-Inflammatory Ingredients: lemon, ginger, turmeric, cinnamon

Ingredients

1 gallon water

8 black tea bags

½ lemon, sliced, rind included

1 inch ginger root, rough chopped

big dash of turmeric

big dash cinnamon

2 tbsp maple syrup (more or less to taste)

Instructions

Bring one gallon of water to a boil. Remove from heat and add all ingredients except for tea bags and return to a boil. Reduce heat and simmer for 10 minutes. Then remove from heat, steep tea bags until cool. Strain into a pitcher and serve over ice. Enjoy!

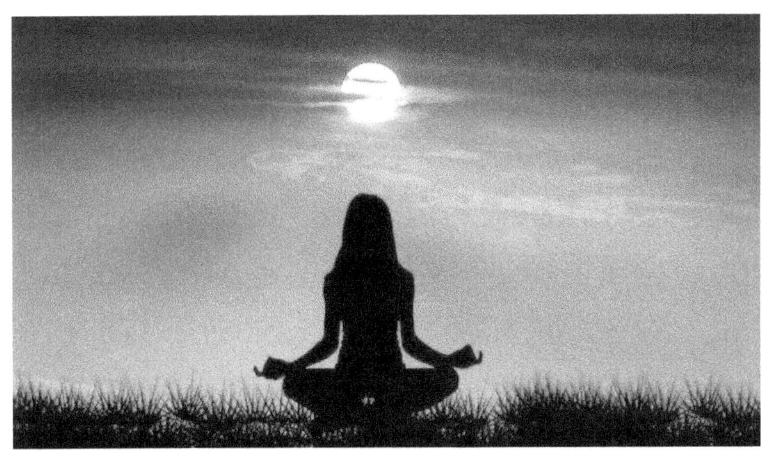

Anti-Inflammatory Lifestyle
Your Body Is Your Temple

I find the science behind nutrition fascinating and I think it can be very helpful to understand how powerful the food we eat is but honestly, it's so simple - eat whole foods!

If you can recognize the ingredients that your food is made of, eat it. Your body will also recognize the food and it will be able to effectively and efficiently convert it into energy and you will be able to feel the difference.

If you clog your body up with toxins, potential allergens, and "foods" that are unrecognizable, imagine the workload you place on it. The liver, gallbladder, and kidneys get clogged up. You literally feel inflamed. You can feel it in your digestion, you may be bloated, you can see it in your skin, and you feel slow, lethargic, and fatigued.

Eat this way consistently and boom, chronic inflammation sets in. Then, the demands on your nervous, immune, circulatory and digestive systems are so much that you are now susceptible to countless diseases and infections. No one wants that and with all of the delicious options out there today, there is no need to. It is as simple as just learning a better way.

It's not that you can never eat another cookie or a side of fries but it is what we do regularly that is most important. Sure, if there is something that makes you happy, go for it but try to eat whole foods most of the time and work to get to a place where you actually want to eat that way. The good news is that eventually you will actually want to eat this way because the unhealthy stuff will not taste nearly as good as it did before. You will start to enjoy healthy foods more and more. It should not feel like punishment or deprivation to eat healthily. It is all about finding a sustainable balance.

Continuing to educate yourself on these topics and understanding how it all works will help you get to a place of joyfully eating a healthy, balanced diet. However, you have to change your mindset first before we can truly change your lifestyles. Mindset is everything.

In addition to the foods that we consume, there are several other lifestyle factors that increase your risk of inflammation. For example, insufficient sleep, stress, and anxiety are known contributors of inflammation. If you are suffering from one, any, or all of these, yoga, and meditation are highly encouraged. They both are well-known remedies that have been very successful with these types of issues. In addition, research suggests that meditation alone may reduce inflammation in the body. Meditation for chronic inflammation consists of a variety of techniques such as paying attention to your breathing and bodily sensations while participating in a physical activity like yoga.

Other risk factors include:

Elevated Cholesterol: Having too much bad cholesterol in our bodies contributes to plaque buildup in our blood vessels. It may also produce an inflammatory response within our bodies which can contribute to even more plaque. This can lead to a blood clot, loosening of the blood clot, and increasing the risk of a stroke and heart attack.

Smoking: Smoking damages blood vessels and our lungs. This damage can cause an inflammatory response. Nicotine alone is inflammatory.

Excessive Drinking: Excessive alcohol consumption is linked to chronic inflammation.

Being Overweight: People that are overweight or suffer from obesity have an increased risk of chronic inflammation. Also, excess belly fat is known to produce a molecule that causes inflammation.

Inactivity: People who are inactive have a greater risk of inflammation. Getting 30 minutes of exercise 3-5 days a week will help reduce inflammation. Taking a brisk walk or bike ride is enough to give you valuable health benefits. Getting regular, moderate exercise is one of the best things you can do for your overall health.

Dehydration: Health professionals have always recommended plenty of fresh drinking water to help manage inflammation. Water in particular because it can help to flush out toxins and other irritants.

Water is a critical element of the body and keeping the body adequately hydrated is essential for optimal function. Even mild dehydration has effects at the cellular level by releasing histamine and Cortisol, which suppress your immune system and causes toxic build up and inflammation.

Inflammation is the body's natural response to irritants as it attempts to eliminate them so drinking plenty of water only makes sense. Water supports the production of lymph that carries the white blood cells throughout the body to fight infections.

Our bodies are made up of approximately 70% water. That water must be continuously replaced. What we replace it with makes a profound difference to our health.

As you work at changing your lifestyle to an anti-inflammatory lifestyle, it is very likely that you will start to notice some positive changes in your body and overall health. An anti-inflammatory lifestyle can lead to better sleep, weight loss, reduced anxiety, lower blood pressure, lower blood sugar, improvement in muscle and joint pain, reduction of digestive issues, and feeling more energetic.

As you can see, there are real, tangible benefits to doing what you can to fight inflammation. You will be healthier, reduce your risk of developing other chronic diseases, and chances are, you will feel better and have more energy.

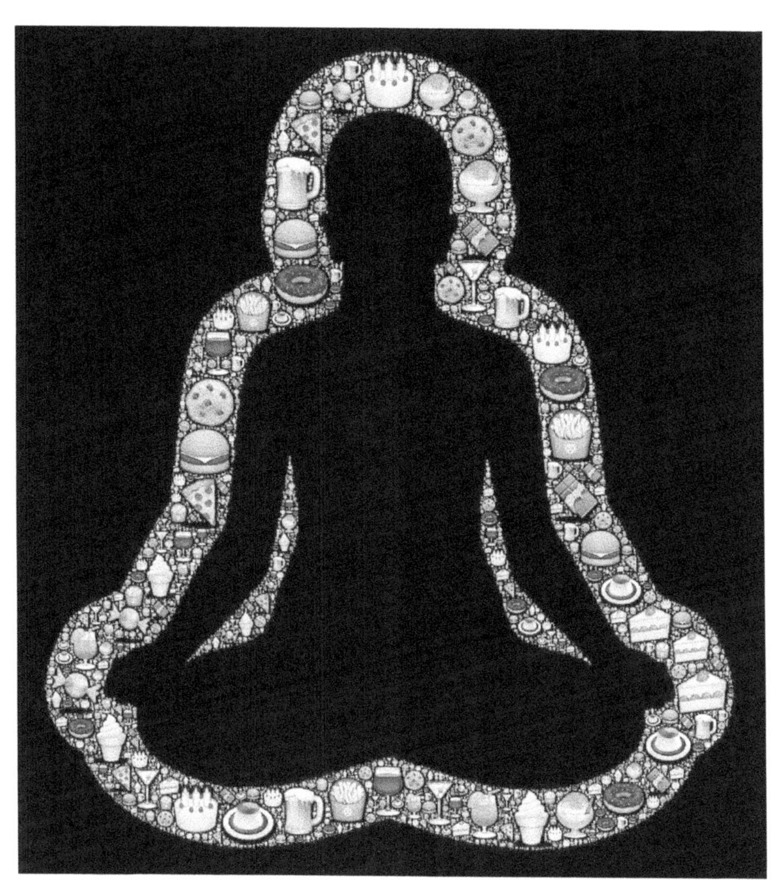

Foods to Avoid

Remember, good health is as much about what you do not eat as it is about what you do eat. Let that sink in.

The foods listed below are just a few of the foods that cause inflammation. Try to avoid or limit these foods as much as possible.

- French fries and other fried foods
- Soda and other sugar-sweetened beverages
- Red meat (burgers, steaks), processed and cured meats, such as hot dogs and lunchmeat
- Margarine, shortening, and lard
- Foods containing trans fats

- Packaged snack foods, like chips
- Processed cheese like velveeta, american cheese slices, cheez whiz, etc.
- White flour items like white pasta, white bread, and pastries

Inflammatory foods are processed or highly refined and they contain a high amount of saturated fats. Processed meats like lunch meats, hot dogs, and fried foods are inflammatory. Refined carbs and simple sugars like white bread, pastries, candy, high fructose corn syrup, soda, and sugar are also inflammatory. They cause blood sugar spikes that trigger inflammation. Over consumption of these foods have been linked to heart disease, diabetes, cancer, and obesity. Moderation is key!

Dairy Products

Dairy products are high in saturated fat but that's not really the issue. The issue is that toxic overload is a root cause of inflammation and dairy products that come from conventional dairy factories are high in toxins which our immune systems must process and eliminate. The toxins in conventional dairy products come in the form of pesticides and antibiotic residue and genetically modified soy used in cattle feed.

I don't know about you, but I have no plans on giving up cheese anytime soon. The solution? Switch to organic dairy products. Grass-fed, pasture-raised organic dairy is the solution.

If you think that dairy might be an inflammation contributor for you, try eliminating it from your diet for a few weeks and see what happens.

Another thing that is important to note here is that dark green leafy vegetables like spinach as well as broccoli and several other fruits and vegetables are excellent sources of calcium.

It is also important to mention that cow's milk is a common allergen and allergies are a cause of inflammation. Milk products are known to stimulate the secretion of cytokines which elicit an inflammatory response.

Eggs & Inflammation

Eggs are tricky when it comes to inflammation and are really very individualized. The arachidonic acid found in egg yolks can contribute to inflammation in the body but, there is currently no evidence that suggests that removing eggs from your diet will prevent inflammation development or improve its symptoms.

The good news is that eggs have been shown to contain compounds that may have anti-inflammatory properties. For this reason, eating two eggs per week as a part of a well-balanced diet is recommended for most adults, including those with inflammatory issues.

For years, eating eggs has been controversial, as they have both good and bad inflammatory properties. Overall, specific research on the effects egg's have on inflammation is limited.

If a person has an egg intolerance or allergy, research shows that they will likely experience an improvement in their inflammatory symptoms by eliminating them from their diet.

However, if you don't have an egg allergy or intolerance, there's currently no research indicating a need to eliminate this nutritious food from your diet. If you are worried that eggs are contributing to your inflammation, you can always try cutting them out for a few weeks to see if you notice any improvements.

Does Gluten Cause Inflammation?

The issue is not necessarily gluten, especially if you don't have an allergy or sensitivity to it. The issue is in the amounts that are being eaten and how wheat looks today in comparison to its original form.

Unless you are allergic to wheat and grains, they do not cause an inflammatory response. Whole-grain consumption has actually been associated with less inflammation and not more.

Numerous studies have pointed to whole grains causing less inflammation in the body so you do not have to be concerned about enjoying healthy, complex carbohydrates in the form of whole grains. However, if you have a wheat intolerance or allergy, or are sensitive to gluten, wheat certainly can cause inflammation.

Remember, you are what you eat. Food is energy. If you eat whole, real food that is organically grown and as local as you can get, it will provide the highest-quality energy and nutrients for you to nourish your body.

Carbohydrates

There are so many misconceptions about carbohydrates. Carbohydrates are necessary to live and they are essential to our health. What determines whether or not a carbohydrate is healthy, is the source. Unfortunately, many people are getting their carbohydrates in the form of overly processed foods which are typically high in refined sugars.

Carbohydrates are a quick source of energy. A good source of carbohydrates can make you feel energized while poor sources can leave you feeling lethargic. It is important to know the difference so you can choose the right carbs to help with your inflammation.

Simple Versus Complex Carbohydrates

Both simple and complex carbs are eventually converted into glucose, the leftovers are converted into glycogen and are either used immediately or stored for energy. The process of how this occurs is a little different for each carbohydrate source.

Simple carbohydrates such as refined sugars and grains are digested quickly causing a spike and consequent crashes in blood sugar levels. If we consistently eat foods that spike our blood sugar, we start to run the risk of decreased insulin sensitivity.

Insulin resistance can lead to conditions related to chronic inflammation such as obesity, heart disease, diabetes, and cancer. Complex carbohydrates are digested more slowly, helping to maintain more stable blood sugar levels.

When choosing carbohydrates from grains, reach for whole-grain options like amaranth, barley, buckwheat, millet, and quinoa. Other good sources of complex carbohydrates include sweet potato, beans, lentils, blueberries, broccoli and oats.

What About Fruit?

The simple carbohydrates in refined foods such as candy bars are the most inflammatory but there are also healthy, anti-inflammatory foods such as fruits and some vegetables that are simple carbohydrates. Unlike candy bars, however, fruits and vegetables also contain fiber and micronutrients that outweigh the cost of the simple sugars.

Fruits and starchy vegetables can be a great source of energy and both are packed with many nutrients. You certainly don't want to eliminate them but just don't over do it and stick to the appropriate serving sizes.

What Foods Are Refined Carbohydrates?

If you're unsure of what refined grains are, think of packaged and frozen desserts, conventional store-bought white bread, processed cookies, cakes, muffins and pastries, processed granola bars, white pasta, and sugary breakfast cereals, frozen pizzas, and basically anything else that can be found on the packaged snack aisle.

Not all of these products contain refined carbohydrates. There definitely are some exceptions. The examples above are just to give you a general idea and most of these conventional type products do contain loads of refined carbohydrates but nowadays, fortunately, there are many unconventional options. It is all about reading the labels and these are the types of foods that you want to pay close attention to.

Processed foods with high amounts of refined sugar include soda, juice, condiments like ketchup and BBQ sauce, pasta sauces, frozen meals, white sugar and processed food with corn syrup or high-fructose corn syrup listed. When you start paying attention to the labels on these types of products, some of you may be shocked to actually find out what is in the products that you have been eating.

If sugar, corn syrup, or high-fructose corn syrup are listed high on the ingredient list, you're looking at added refined sugars.

The best sources of carbohydrates are whole plant foods. Whole food sources of complex carbohydrates also provide important minerals, vitamins, and fiber that make you feel full longer than refined carbohydrates, helping you to maintain healthy body weight.

What About Fiber?

Fiber is a super important type of complex carbohydrate. It improves the body's ability to utilize nutrients and balance blood sugar levels. It also plays an important role in gut bacteria, maintaining regular bowel movements, and supports healthy intestines.

Nutritional guidelines suggest that we get at least 30 grams of fiber per day but it is common for people to get less than half of that. This can be improved by including more vegetables, whole grains, beans, and fruits in your diet.

Diets low in fiber can cause constipation, IBC, and diverticulitis. Conditions that are either a consequence or a cause of chronic inflammation.

What About Protein?

Protein is made up of amino acids. We use amino acids for cell growth, metabolism, immune defense, and repair. Protein is an essential nutrient for healing. I am not going to go too deep into protein but some of the healthier choices you can make to get the best protein into your anti-inflammatory diet are:

- Seeds and Nuts
- Legumes
- Beans
- Cooked seed grains such as quinoa
- Organic, free range, grass-fed meats
- Eggs, free-range, seed fed animals
- Organic dairy

What About Fats?

Fats play a big roleinflammation. By reducing the number of processed foods you eat, you will naturally reduce inflammation because processed foods typically contain pro-inflammatory refined oils. This includes oils like vegetable oil, corn oil, sunflower oil, and safflower oil. You should try to completely eliminate any trans fats in your diet, most commonly listed on packaging as partially hydrogenated oils.

Instead of getting our dietary fats from the oils added to processed foods, we should focus on adding high-quality fats from foods such as avocados, nuts, seeds, and natural nut butter.

We need dietary fat to maintain vital body functions, support cell growth, and inhibit excessive fat storage. Rather than being concerned about how much fat you consume, you should pay attention to the type of fat you consume.

Three Types of Fats

Fatty acids fall into one of three major categories:

- **Saturated Fatty Acids (SFAs)** – Most are from dairy products, red meat, poultry, and processed foods.
- **Monounsaturated Fatty Acids (MUFAs)** – Are found in oils such as olive oil as well as avocado. Monounsaturated Fatty Acids are known as the "good fat".
- **Essential Polyunsaturated Fatty Acids (PUFAs omega-3 and omega-6)**

These are essential fatty acids that the body needs for brain function and cell growth. Our bodies do not make essential fatty acids, so we must get them from food.

Before we get into the essential fatty acids. Let's take a quick look at saturated and monounsaturated fatty acids. Most people think that saturated fats are bad for you and this is true to a certain extent but only if you consume excessive amounts of them.

For example, a high intake of saturated fatty acids from grain-fed farm animals contributes to inflammation. They also compete with the essential fatty acids, omega-3 and omega-6 for metabolic enzymes, increase levels of pro-inflammatory chemicals, and congest the liver.

A moderate amount of saturated fats can be put to good use in a healthy body. Excessive intake of any fat can be detrimental if your liver and gallbladder are congested. Again remember, balance of all dietary fats, eaten in moderation is key.

Eliminating Trans Fats

Trans fats are made through a process called hydrogenation in which an otherwise healthy monounsaturated fat is exposed to heat, turning it into a solid. Trans fats are used heavily in processed foods for their ability to extend the shelf life of foods.

Hydrogenated oils are found in everything from processed peanut butter and cheeses to low-fat "health foods" and many of the cookies, crackers and other processed food you would find in a traditional grocery store. Make sure you read ingredients lists and look for hydrogenated or partially hydrogenated oils and try to eliminate anything containing those from your diet.

Cooking Oils

One of the problems with oils in the typical American diet today is that unstable oils are being used to fry and cook foods on high heat. It is common to fry foods with olive oil but this damages the oil. Avocado oil and coconut oil both have high smoke points and are the better for higher heat cooking but never allow them to reach their smoke point. The smoke point of an oil is the temperature at which it stops shimmering and starts smoking. The smoke point is also called the burning point of oil.

The Omega-3 to Omega-6 Imbalance

The intake of vegetable oils has increased substantially over the years. Overconsumption of these processed oils has thrown off the ratio of omega-3 to omega-6 in the typical American diet. With people including more and more processed and refined foods as well as grain-fed, conventional animal meats, the ratio is more disproportionate than ever.

People are now consuming as much as 25 times more omega-6s than they should be getting. Many health authorities believe that the overconsumption of omega-6 is contributing to the increasing rate of inflammatory conditions today.

Omega-3 and omega-6 essential fatty acids are the most anti-inflammatory fats. Both fats, when consumed in the proper ratio, from high-quality sources have powerful anti-inflammatory properties. They support cardiovascular health, lubricate joints and skin, boost the metabolism, support healthy immune and nervous systems and help balance hormones.

Where Do Omega-6s Come From?

Omega-6 fatty acids are much more common in the typical American Diet. They are in corn oil, peanut oil, soybean oil, canola oil, and sunflower oil. All of these oils are used in cooking and used heavily in processed foods.

The poor quality of omega-6 fatty acids in American diets today not only decreases their power as an anti-inflammatory but actually makes them inflammatory. Not only that, the excess of omega-6 in our diets today makes it difficult for the body to use the enzyme needed to convert foods like nuts and seeds into usable omega-3.

One of the reasons that omega-6 becomes inflammatory is that essential fatty acids are extremely sensitive to high heat, light, and free radicals. When those sources of omega-6 fatty acids are used in frying, cooking, hydrogenation, and refined for use in processed foods, they become damaged. Damaged essential fatty acids are really hard on our bodies, particularly on the liver.

The best thing you can do to improve your diet if you are consuming a substantial amount of omega-6 is to work towards eliminating these sources from your diet. You can switch to avocado, olive, and sesame seed oils to replace refined vegetable oils and cut out all over-processed foods in your diet.

Make sure you are using raw, unrefined oils and if you do cook with oils, use oils that can handle higher temperatures such as coconut or avocado oil.

Overconsumption

While most people are over-consuming omega-6 fatty acids, omega-3s are vastly under-consumed.

Omega-3 deficiency can lead to:

- excess inflammation
- asthma
- diabetes
- arthritis
- hormone imbalances
- cancer
- skin conditions such as eczema and psoriasis

You want at least a 2:1 ratio of omega-3 versus omega-6 fatty acids in your diet. Omega-9s are important too and those come from monounsaturated fats found in foods like avocado, macadamia nuts, and olive oil.

Omega-3s For Inflammation

Omega-3s are really important for our overall health. They can prevent cardiovascular disease, they nourish the brain and nervous tissue, reduce symptoms of anxiety, depression, and joint pain, and have overall powerful anti-inflammatory properties.

Problems are likely to occur when we eat too many omega-6s and not enough omega-3s. When this happens, omega-3s can't do their job. Omega 3's are great for reducing inflammation. All it takes is just being aware of your intake - it's easy to increase the amount of omega-3 in your diet.

Salmon, walnuts, chia seeds, hemp seeds, and flax seeds are all high in omega 3 essential fatty acids.

Micronutrients

Micronutrients include things like phytonutrients, antioxidants, vitamins, and minerals are a big part of eating an anti-inflammatory diet.

To ensure you are eating a wide range of phytonutrients, eat vegetables in a variety of colors. The best colors to look for when it comes to promoting anti-inflammation are dark blues and purples such as blueberries and blackberries, and bright reds, yellows, and oranges like bell peppers, squash, and sweet potatoes. And the color of dark green in the form of dark leafy greens like chard, kale, and spinach.

You can also drink white and green tea to increase the amount of phytonutrients you are consuming. Just remember that these teas contain caffeine so they should be avoided if you are sensitive to it. Also, keep in mind that caffeine is a diuretic so make sure to drink plenty of water.

Hydration & Inflammation

We have already briefly discussed the importance of hydration so I am not going to go too deep into it but it is really pretty simple. Chronic dehydration contributes to chronic inflammation.

Drink water steadily throughout the day and drink long before you feel thirsty to prevent ever being dehydrated. Dehydration negatively affects every system of the body. It slows digestion, metabolism drops, heart rate and blood pressure increase, and mental and physical abilities are reduced. It also causes constipation, indigestion, poor circulation, local inflammation, joint pain and muscle stiffness, and loss of flexibility.

When you feel like you are having a dip in energy levels, reach for a glass of water before anything else. Drinking coffee or sugary drinks as an energy source is only going to worsen the problem. To prevent chronic dehydration, drink more water, aiming for 8 to 12 glasses a day. Cut back on coffee and soda, and reduce the amount of refined sugars, table salt, and processed foods you eat.

Hidden Sources

With so many healthy food options, it can be hard to choose the best and most healthy products but the ingredients list does not lie. Do not be fooled by the labeling and sales gimmicks. Sure the labels can be helpful when determining which product to purchase but they do not always provide the whole picture. For example, a product may be labeled as vegetarian but that does not mean that it is healthy. There are many vegetarian products out there that contain unhealthy ingredients. What you really need to be looking at is what the ingredients are. Are the ingredients whole food nutrients? Or, is the list of ingredients full of artificial and processed ingredients that you do not even recognize? Unfortunately, we often come across these hidden ingredients without even knowing it. The problem is that for some of us, they can trigger issues like inflammation.

No more wondering if your "healthy" foods are actually healthy. Now you can be your own advocate. Always read the list of ingredients and choose products with a short and an easy to recognize list of ingredients.

So what foods commonly contain these hidden inflammatory ingredients? You may be surprised. Some of the most common ingredients are:

- High-fructose corn syrup
- MSG
- Refined oils like soybean oil, canola oil, and vegetable oil
- Artificial sweeteners and sugar alcohols like sucralose, xylitol, and aspartame
- Sodium nitrate

- Trans fats and partially hydrogenated oils
- Sodium nitrate
- Carrageenan

Have you even taken a look at the ingredients in your favorite snack? We are going to review some common foods and snack foods that often come off as healthy but in fact, they are actually filled with junk.

There are healthy options that are made with wholesome nutrients but unfortunately, this is not the case for many of the typical store-bought products.

Trail Mix and Granola

Unfortunately, it is not uncommon for store bought trail mix and granola to be loaded with sodium and sugar. A lot of the well known brands roast the nuts in hydrogenated oils. They also often have sweetened dried fruit and other sugary additives.

The Solution: Make your own trail mix or granola. Or find products without hydrogenated oil that are made with raw ingredients.

Flavored Yogurt

It is very common for this "healthy" snack or breakfast product to be loaded with artificial sweeteners and other unhealthy ingredients. High fructose corn syrup is one of them you see often in yogurts. Don't let the sugar free label fool you. Try to avoid flavored yogurts unless they are flavored with natural honey and/or other whole foods.

The Solution: Find brands that offer products without artificial sweeteners and other artificial ingredients. There are healthy options, you just have to find them. Another solution is to buy whole plain yogurt and add fruit and nuts to it. The fruit sweetens it naturally.

Frozen Yogurts

Sure, frozen yogurts are usually healthier than ice cream but again, not all of them. Many have artificial fillers, artificial sugars, and sugar alcohols. A lot of these artificial fillers, sugars, and sugar alcohols are inflammatory triggers.

The Solution: Again, you just have to read the labels and look for those artificial unhealthy ingredients mentioned before. Stick to products with minimal and whole ingredients. There are almost as many of these products as there are of those unhealthier frozen yogurts. If you can't find any, you may be shopping at the wrong stores.

Chips and Crackers

Some chips and crackers may be labeled as healthy but it is important to do your homework and read the labels with these savory snacks.

Look for those hidden ingredients. In products like these you might see sugars, vegetable oil, and high sodium content.

The Solution: A good rule of thumb is that healthier products typically have much fewer ingredients than unhealthy products. Also, you should be able to pronounce the names of the ingredients. There are exceptions, but usually the names of the ingredients are recognizable words that you can pronounce.

Deli Meat

We have already touched on deli meat a little but in addition to the nitrates and sodium, these products often contain sugars such as dextrose which can also trigger inflammation.

The Solution: Choose products that do not contain these ingredients. Natural, organic, grass fed products. As mentioned before, you can get these from the grocers deli, organic products, and/or if you have one, your local Farmers Market.

Veggie Burgers

Shocking but true, there are several brands out there using "healthy" on their veggie burger labels but contain unhealthy ingredients. These hidden ingredients might be hydrogenated oils like soybean or canola, fillers, and high amounts of sodium. But there are many healthy options available.

The Solution: Read the labels! Look for veggie burgers with natural whole food ingredients. For example vegetables, beans, lentils, and quinoa, not soy protein or other processed ingredients.

Protein Bars

Most of us choose these bars as a healthy snack or breakfast that we can take on the go. We think that they are loaded with nutrients that are good for us but often that is not the case. Many of them are pretty much the same as eating a candy bar. High fructose corn syrup, saturated fats, and refined oils.

The Solution: There are many really healthy options. Again, read the labels. These bars tend to be expensive. You certainly do not want to be thinking you are having a healthy snack, when you are actually eating a candy bar. Choose the brands with wholesome ingredients.

Salad Dressing

Again, main ingredients are always listed first in all packaging. Many salad dressings have sugar, hydrogenated and canola oil in the beginning of their list of ingredients as their main ingredients. They are also often high in sodium and other inflammatory ingredients.

The Solution: Fortunately, healthy salad dressing options are becoming more and more readily available. They are usually located in the refrigerated section of the grocery store near the produce. It is also very easy to make your own and you will find recipes for several later in the book.

Whole Grain Cereal

We all know that traditional cereals are typically loaded with sugars and often synthetic dyes but most people would not expect to find them in whole

grain cereal. Most of these products are actually made with wholesome ingredients and rich in fiber but there are a few that are not.

The Solution: Read the list of ingredients and look for cereals with wholesome ingredients that have less than 8 grams of sugar per serving.

Instant Oatmeal

No doubt that oatmeal is a great healthy option but only when it does not contain a lot of artificial ingredients. Often instant oatmeal is loaded with sugar. It may seem convenient and again not all instant oatmeal is bad, you just have to do your homework and read the list of ingredients.

The Solution: Choose instant oatmeal from a wholesome source that is unsweetened. Or, make your own overnight oats and sweeten it with real fruit.

Pasta Sauce

Many pasta sauces are loaded with inflammatory ingredients like refined oils and sugars. Fortunately, there are many healthy options.

The Solution: Look for pasta sauce with wholesome ingredients like olive oil, real tomatoes and other vegetables, and herbs.

Do Nightshades Cause Inflammation?

I have been hearing a lot of questions lately about nightshade vegetables and their relation to inflammation. Nightshades are a family of plants that include tomatoes, eggplant, potatoes, peppers, and tobacco. Nightshades are unique because they contain small amounts of alkaloids.

Alkaloids are chemicals that are mainly found in plants. For something to be considered an alkaloid, it must contain nitrogen and affect the human body, usually from a medicinal perspective.

While some alkaloids have positive effects on human health, others can affect them negatively. For example, the chemicals found in tobacco can cause cancer.

The alkaloid found in nightshades is solanine. It functions as an insecticide while the plant is growing.

Eating too much solanine can make you feel bad. When potatoes turn green, they have more alkaloids in them, and they can taste bitter. That is why people usually recommend throwing out green and/or sprouting potatoes. If you eat green potatoes, you may get sick to your stomach with nausea or diarrhea. You can also get a fever or headache. Although normally, potatoes and other nightshade vegetables have an acceptable amount of alkaloids in them.

Tomatoes contain more alkaloids in the stem and vine than in the fruit. Studies show that as tomatoes mature, the amount of alkaloids in the part eaten decreases. So, it is unlikely to eat too many alkaloids from tomatoes, especially if you avoid unripe, green tomatoes.

How do you know if nightshades are bad for you? Experts recommend eliminating them from your diet for a few weeks. Then, reintroduce them and see how you feel. If you feel worse after reintroduction, you may have a sensitivity to nightshades.

Whether or not there is any conclusive evidence about nightshades and inflammation, you should never eat any foods that make you feel bad, or that worsen any condition you have.

It is important to note that there is no hard evidence that suggests that nightshade vegetables are bad for your health. There has been some preliminary research that shows that these vegetables may not be the best for people with certain inflammatory and auto-immune conditions like arthritis or inflammatory bowel disease. Nightshades do not cause inflammation directly. However, they can increase inflammation that is already present.

Benefits of Nightshades

There are nutrients in nightshades that can be good for your health. They contain antioxidants that protect cells from damage due to stress.

For example, anthocyanin, the antioxidant that gives eggplant its purple color can reduce the risk of developing cancer, diabetes, and infections.

The antioxidant lycopene, found in tomatoes, may decrease the risk of some types of cancer and heart disease.

Nightshades also contain vitamins and minerals that contribute to good health, like Vitamin A and Vitamin C. Eating one bell pepper, for example, gives you your daily recommended amount of Vitamin C and also has anti-inflammatory benefits.

Consuming Nightshades

If you are concerned about high alkaloid content in nightshade vegetables but still want to benefit from including them in your diet, there are a few things you can try:

- In potatoes, the highest concentration of alkaloids is in the skin. One study showed that skinning potatoes before cooking removed up to 70 percent of the alkaloids.
- Store potatoes in a dark, cool place to prevent them from producing more alkaloids before you eat them.

Eating Out

Eating out is less tricky than you might think. Now that you know what you should be eating and what you should avoid, just follow the same guidelines. Below you find some ideas for meals at different types of restaurants.

Asian Restaurants

The first question that comes up with Asian restaurants is "can I have sushi?". While you do want to stay away from the fried options, white rice, and cream sauces, there are a ton of anti-inflammatory options. Sushi ingredients like tuna, mackerel, salmon, seaweed, vegetables (including pickled vegetables), brown rice, and wasabi are all anti-inflammatory.

Italian Restaurants

Great options at Italian restaurants would be:

- Whole wheat pasta served with a vegetable marinara sauce or olive oil.
- Baked or grilled chicken or fish with a side of veggies. Make sure to request it with no cream sauce.
- Seafood stew (or cioppino). If it is prepared with a cream sauce, ask if it can be replaced with something like tomatoes in a wine sauce.

Greek Restaurants

Greek restaurants are a great choice for those on an anti- inflammatory diet because they usually offer so many options that are delicious and anti-inflammatory. It is pretty safe to say that you can have most things offered at

Greek restaurants. Just remember the foods to avoid and you will be fine.

Indian Cuisine

Indian food is another great option because so many of the spices used are anti-inflammatory (turmeric, clove, cinnamon, ginger).

You want to avoid dishes that contain cream. Try ordering curry or dal (lentil or garbanzo-based).

Tandoori is a great option. Try chicken or fish tandoori.

What About Fast Food?

While it is best to avoid fast food, sometimes you have no other choice. And, fortunately, more and more restaurants are offering healthier choices. If you are fortunate enough to have a Wendy's, El Pollo Loco, or similar type of restaurant, these establishments have some of the most healthy fast food options.

Some general suggestions when making your selections:

- Skip the bacon, french fries, and sauce.
- Avoid soda and milkshakes.
- If you get a burger, don't eat the bread unless there's a whole wheat option.
- Order grilled instead of fried.

- Choose a salad with a vinaigrette & olive oil-type dressing.

Good Meal Choice Examples:

- A fajita with grilled chicken or seafood topped with lettuce and tomatoes or other veggies.
- A spinach salad with grilled chicken, veggies, nuts, and low-fat/vinaigrette type dressing.
- Taco salad with black beans, avocado, chicken, and salsa.

Meal Delivery Services

I wanted to include this section because I realize many people want to eat healthy meals but simply lack the time. In addition, not everyone knows how or likes to cook. That is where healthy meal delivery services come in. These convenient services offer prepared meals for different types of diets. In the next section there's a list of services that offer Anti-Inflammatory meals. Below I've listed a few general guidelines to follow when ordering from these convenient services.

- Carefully review the ingredients and nutritional information.
- Some meal services allow for customization while others do not.
- Most of these services offer single servings that only need to be heated

but some do require a little time to prepare.

Meal Delivery Services

The Good Kitchen

www.thegoodkitchen.com

This service creates and prepares tasty meals according to your unique needs, including an anti-inflammatory diet. All you need to do is heat up your meal and enjoy it, safe in the knowledge that it's as nutritious as it is tasty.

Urban Remedy

https://urbanremedy.com/meal-plans-cleanses/anti-inflammation-meal-plan-guide/

Urban Remedy offers an anti-inflammatory meal plan that delivers 3 days of organic, non-GMO, plant-based nutrition that eliminates the top inflammatory foods common to the

American diet like gluten, refined sugar, caffeine, processed meats, and dairy. It features some of the most nutrient-rich plant-based recipes to satisfy all your cravings. Low glycemic, organic goodness chock full of antioxidants and phytonutrients to support being your best self.

The Custom Plate

https://thecustomplate.com
The Custom Plate offers an affordable anti-inflammatory meal delivery subscription.

BistroMD -

www.bistromd.com
BistroMD has a great anti-inflammatory meal delivery service. They offer signature/customized meal subscriptions that are prepared by dieticians and chefs to cater to your unique ingredients.

Factor 75

https://www.factor75.com/

Healthy eating, made easy. Fresh, ready-made meals delivered to your doorstep. A new menu of 30+ dietitian-designed options every week.

Fresh N' Lean

https://www.freshnlean.com/mediterranean-diet-meal-delivery/

Enjoy fresh, chef-cooked meals made the Mediterranean Diet way. Packed with anti-inflammatory whole foods and healthy fats that support longevity and heart health. Choose your meals. Get them delivered. Ready-to-eat in just 3 minutes.

Anti-Inflammatory Meal Kits

A meal kit is a subscription food service where a company sends customers pre-portioned and sometimes partially-prepared food ingredients and recipes to prepare home cooked meals.

Purple Carrot

https://www.purplecarrot.com/weekly-menu/meal-kits

Easy recipes and ingredients delivered right to your door. Make healthy meals that you will love.

Sunbasket

https://sunbasket.com/

Delicious meals made from farm fresh, organic ingredients.

Quick recipes, ready in minutes, designed for busy people, delivered to your door. Meal Planning Made Easy - Put meal planning on autopilot to eat well all week.

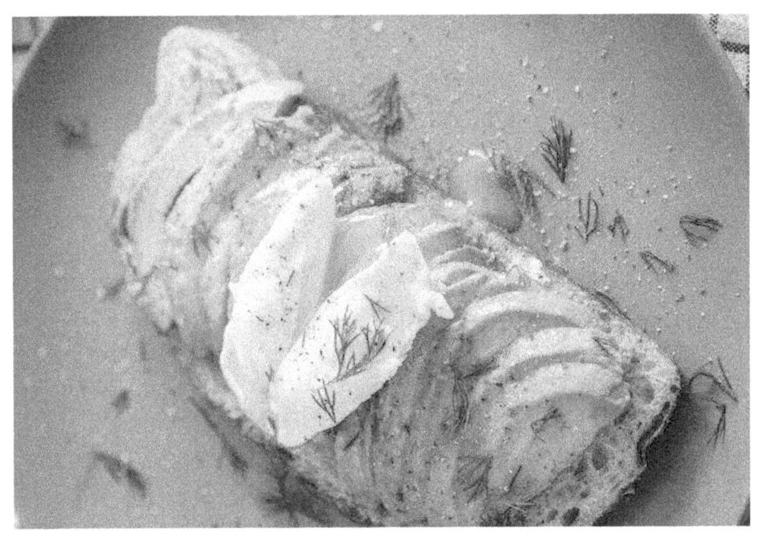

Breakfast Recipes

Good Morning Egg & Avocado Toast

This Egg & Avocado Toast is delicious and is so healthy. It's the perfect way to start the day. Enjoy!

Anti-Inflammatory Ingredients: avocado, pepper, sesame seeds, dill

Servings: 2
Time: 20 minutes

Ingredients

2 eggs

2 slices whole wheat bread

1 avocado

⅛ tsp sea salt

⅛ tsp ground black pepper

1 Tbsp grated organic white cheddar cheese

⅛ tsp black sesame seeds

Top with fresh dill

Instructions

- In the first step, we will be soft boiling the eggs. Bring a few inches of water to a boil in a deep saucepan. When the water reaches a boil, lower the heat to medium-high and slowly lower the eggs into the water using a spoon, one at a time.
- For a runny yolk, cook for 6 minutes. Cook one minute longer if you prefer a more firm yolk.
- Remove the egg carefully with a spoon and place it directly into a bowl of ice-cold water. Let the eggs sit in the cold water for 2 minutes.
- Remove the shells from the eggs.
- Toast the bread and set aside.
- Slice the avocado and then spread slices on toast.

- Sprinkle with sea salt and black pepper.
- Place the eggs on top of each piece of avocado toast and gently slice open, spreading it to cover the entire piece of toast.
- Sprinkle with organic shredded cheese, black sesame seeds, and dill. Yum!

Petite Mushroom Spinach Quiche

These three ingredients go together heavenly. What I really love about them is that they freeze well. Make an extra batch and freeze them to have a quick and healthy meal for later.

Anti-Inflammatory Ingredients: extra-virgin olive oil, mushrooms, onion, garlic, thyme, and spinach

Servings: 6
Time: 1 hour

Ingredients

2 Tbsp extra virgin olive oil

8 oz fresh mixed wild mushrooms sliced

1 cup thinly sliced yellow onion

1 Tbsp minced garlic

2 tsp minced fresh thyme

1 (5 oz) package fresh spinach, coarsely chopped

8 large eggs

⅔ cup whole milk

2 tsp healthy Dijon mustard

½ tsp salt

½ tsp ground pepper

¾ cup shredded Gruyère cheese

Instructions

- Preheat the oven to 325 degrees F.
- Heat extra virgin olive oil in a large saute pan, on medium-high.
- Add mushrooms, and cook until browned on the bottom, about 4 minutes. Stir and continue to cook, stirring occasionally, until browned all over, about 5 minutes.
- Add sliced onion, stir and cook until they begin to soften, about 4 minutes.

- Add garlic and thyme, stir and cook for about 2 minutes.
- Add spinach, continue to stir, cook until just wilted, about 2 minutes. Remove from heat.
- Whisk eggs, milk, Dijon, salt, and pepper in a large bowl.
- Add cheese and mushroom mixture.
- Spray a 12-cup muffin pan with extra virgin olive oil. Pour the mixture into the 12 cups of the muffin pan, and distribute evenly (you can place muffin tins in the pan cups if you prefer, it's optional).
- Bake, uncovered for 30 minutes.
- Remove from the pan and serve immediately.
- **Note:** These freeze well. Make an extra batch and freeze them to have a quick and healthy breakfast later.

Creamy Strawberry and Walnut Greek Yogurt

This healthy anti-inflammatory breakfast is super easy and quick to prepare. Make it with your favorite berries. What a great way to start the day!

Anti-inflammatory Ingredients: berries, walnuts

Servings: 1
Time: 5 minutes

Ingredients

½ cup nonfat plain Greek yogurt
¼ cup sliced fresh strawberries
2 Tbsp walnuts

Instructions

Place yogurt in a bowl and top with strawberries and walnuts. Voila - quick, easy, delicious healthy breakfast.

Golden Milk

Also known as haldi doodh, golden milk is a delicious traditional Indian drink known for its healing anti-inflammatory properties. I have placed it in the breakfast section, but it's great any time of the day. Enjoy

Servings: 2
Time: 5 minutes

Ingredients

1 ½ cups coconut milk
1 ½ cups almond milk
1 ½ tsp ground turmeric
¼ tsp ground ginger
¼ tsp ground cinnamon
1 Tbsp coconut oil (optional)
1 pinch ground black pepper
1 Tbsp raw honey (optional)

Instructions

- In a medium pot, add coconut milk, almond milk, turmeric, ginger, cinnamon, coconut oil, black pepper, and honey.

- Whisk ingredients to combine over medium heat for 5 minutes without boiling - whisk frequently.

- Remove from heat and serve immediately.

Notes: Any leftovers can be stored covered in the refrigerator for 2-3 days.

Banana Nut Pancakes

I can't think of a better way to start a weekend morning than with banana nut pancakes. Put on Jack Johnson's Banana Pancakes song and make these delicious pancakes. This is a sure way to get off to a great start to the rest of your day. Enjoy!

Anti-Inflammatory Ingredients: cinnamon, banana, walnuts, and extra virgin olive oil

Servings: 6
Time: 20 minutes

Ingredients

1 cup whole wheat flour

2 tsp baking powder

¼ tsp salt

¼ tsp cinnamon

1 large banana, very ripe, mashed

1 cup 1% milk

3 large egg whites

2 tsp extra virgin olive oil

1 tsp vanilla

2 Tbsp chopped walnuts

Extra virgin olive oil cooking spray

Instructions

- Mix all dry ingredients in a bowl. Beat the egg whites until fluffy.
- Combine milk, oil, vanilla, and mashed bananas in a bowl and mix until smooth. Add the egg whites and mix.
- Combine wet ingredients with the dry and mix well with a spoon until there are no more dry spots.
- Heat a large nonstick skillet on medium heat.
- Spray with olive oil to lightly coat and pour 1/4 cup of pancake batter.

- When the pancake starts to bubble and the edges begin to set, flip the pancakes.
- Repeat with the remainder of the batter.

Cha Cha Chia Pudding

This chia pudding is fantastic and super healthy! Enjoy!

Anti-Inflammatory Ingredients: Tofu, Chia Seeds, Almonds, Blueberries

Servings: 1
Time: 10 minutes

Ingredients

375 ml Almond Milk

4 oz Soft Tofu

½ tsp Pure Almond Extract

¼ cup Chia Seeds

¼ cup Sliced Almonds

1 cup Blueberries

Instructions

- Add almond milk, tofu, and extract to a blender or food processor. Then blend until smooth.
- Pour mixture into a large/medium size bowl, add chia seeds, stir to mix well, and let sit for 10 minutes.
- Heat a small skillet to medium-low heat, add almond slices, and continuously stir until lightly toasted. Remove from heat and set aside.
- Add blueberries to the chia mixture. Refrigerate chia pudding until chilled. Top with toasted almonds and serve.

Raspberry Parfait

Packed with chia seeds, this super healthy Raspberry Parfait is perfect for breakfast or dessert. It's quick, easy, and simple to make.

Anti-Inflammatory Ingredients:
raspberries, chia seeds, cinnamon

Servings: 2
Time: 10 minutes

Ingredients

½ cup fresh raspberries

2 Tbsp chia seeds

1 tsp maple syrup or raw honey

Pinch of cinnamon

16 oz plain yogurt

Fresh fruit of your choice

Instructions

- Place the raspberries in a medium-small size mixing bowl. Mash the berries until they reach a jam-like consistency with the back of a fork. Add the chia seeds, honey, and cinnamon to the bowl. Continue to mash until all of the ingredients are totally combined and mixed well. Set aside.

- Place a layer of yogurt in the bottom of a medium-sized glass or jar. Top with a layer of the raspberry chia mixture. Finish with an additional layer of yogurt. Garnish with fresh sliced fruit and an extra drizzle of maple syrup, if you'd like. Enjoy!

Pecan Banana Oats

Need an easy, deliciously healthy recipe that you can grab on the go or take to work? This is perfect for that and absolutely delicious! Just put it in a jar with a lid.

Anti-Inflammatory Ingredients: banana, chia seeds, pecans, figs, pomegranate seeds

Servings: 2
Time: 15 minutes (plus 6 hours in fridge or overnight)

Ingredients

1 cup old-fashioned rolled oats

1 ½ cups milk

2 ripe bananas, mashed

¼ cup plain Greek yogurt

2 Tbsp unsweetened coconut flakes,
toasted
2 Tbsp honey
1 Tbsp chia seeds
2 tsp vanilla extract
¼ tsp flaked sea salt

Topping

Banana slices
Roasted pecans
Fig halves
Drizzle of honey
Pomegranate seeds

Instructions

- Place the oats, milk, bananas, Greek yogurt, unsweetened coconut flakes, honey, chia seeds, vanilla extract, and sea salt in a medium size bowl and stir until all ingredients are combined.

- Divide the mixture between 2 small bowls or glass jars.
- Cover and refrigerate for at least 6 hours or overnight.
- Stir, heat up if desired, and top with banana slices, roasted pecans, and fig halves. Drizzle with honey and sprinkle with pomegranate seeds. Delicious!

Wake Me Up Mocha Cherry Smoothie

This Mocha Cherry Smoothie is delicious and it's quick and easy to make.

Anti-Inflammatory Ingredients: cocoa powder, cherries, banana, dark chocolate

Servings: 2
Time: 10 minutes

Ingredients

1 cup frozen unsweetened pitted dark sweet cherries

1 cup unsweetened chocolate almond milk

6 oz vanilla fat-free Greek yogurt

½ medium banana

2 Tbsp unsweetened cocoa powder

2 Tbsp almond butter

1 tsp instant espresso coffee powder

1 tsp vanilla

2 cups ice cubes

1 Tbsp dark chocolate shavings (make sure 70%)

Instructions

- Add cherries, almond milk, Greek yogurt, banana, cocoa powder, almond butter, espresso coffee powder, and vanilla to a blender and blend until smooth.
- Serve in two glasses topped with chocolate shavings and banana slices.

Tip: Peel the remaining banana half, wrap tightly in plastic wrap, then in foil. Freeze for next time.

Tropical Ginger Smoothie

This festive smoothie is packed with anti-inflammatory goodness. What a treat!

Anti-Inflammatory Ingredients: ginger, pineapple, flax seed, turmeric, cinnamon

Servings: 1
Time: 5 minutes

Ingredients

1 tsp fresh ginger (about 1 inch, peeled)
8 oz coconut milk (can use nut milk of choice)
1 frozen banana (cut into thirds)
1 cup frozen pineapple chunks
1 tsp ground flaxseed
½ tsp ground turmeric
Pinch ground cinnamon
2-3 ice cubes (optional)

Instructions

Put peeled ginger into a blender and pulse for 5-10 seconds until finely chopped. Add coconut milk, banana, pineapple, flax seed, turmeric, cinnamon, and ice (optional) then blend on high for 2 minutes. Pour into a glass and enjoy!

Sweet Potato Hash

This savory Sweet Potato Hash is filled with anti-inflammatory ingredients and is one of my favorites. Enjoy!

Anti-Inflammatory Ingredients: sweet potatoes, red onion, garlic, extra virgin olive oil, pepper, and green onions

Servings: 3
Time: 45 minutes

Ingredients

3 sweet potatoes, cubed
½ red onion, diced
1 clove garlic, minced
1 Tbsp extra virgin olive oil
½ tsp sea salt
¼ tsp black pepper
2 green onions, sliced for topping

Instructions

- Preheat oven to 425 degrees F and line a rimmed baking sheet with parchment paper.
- Add the cubed sweet potatoes, red onion, and garlic to the baking sheet.
- Drizzle the ingredients on the baking sheet with extra virgin olive oil, sprinkle with sea salt and pepper then toss to coat well.
- Spread all of the ingredients on the baking sheet into an even layer.
- Bake for 25-30 minutes, tossing once halfway through. When it is fully cooked, the potatoes will be golden and tender in the middle. Test with a fork before serving.

Tofu Breakfast Burritos

Rise and shine with these delicious breakfast burritos. Packed with anti-inflammatory ingredients, this healthy, hearty breakfast will keep you going all morning long. Yum!

Anti-Inflammatory Ingredients: extra virgin olive oil, tofu, pepper, black beans, avocado, pico do gallo

Servings: 4
Time: 15 minutes

Ingredients

2 Tbsp extra virgin olive oil
2 cups crumbled extra firm tofu
1 pinch salt
1 pinch pepper

2 pinches AI spice blend

4 whole wheat tortillas

1 cup cooked black beans

1 avocado

1 cup pico de gallo

Instructions

- Heat the tortillas according to the package instructions.
- In a sauté pan, heat olive oil. Add tofu, salt, pepper, and turmeric. Cook for about 5 minutes.
- Place a portion of tofu, beans, avocados, and pico in the center of the tortillas and fold sides in, and roll to close. Serve.

Note: Some tofu comes in water. If yours did, drain and press with paper towels. Tofu can be crumbled by hand, or pulsed in a food processor. Either way will be fine.

Carrot Cake
Breakfast Cookies

Cookies for breakfast? Yes, please! These Carrot Cake Breakfast Cookies are a nice treat for breakfast, a snack, or dessert. Enjoy!

Anti-Inflammatory Ingredients: cinnamon, nutmeg, ginger, clove, carrots, walnuts

Servings: 12 - 14 cookies
Time: 1 hour

Ingredients

1 cup instant oats

¾ cup whole wheat flour

1 ½ tsp baking powder

1 ½ tsp ground cinnamon

¼ tsp ground nutmeg

¼ tsp salt

2 Tbsp coconut oil

1 large egg white

1 tsp vanilla

¼ cup pure maple syrup

5 Tbsp nonfat milk

¾ cup fresh grated carrots (peel before shredding)

Instructions

- Add the oats, flour, baking powder, cinnamon, nutmeg, and salt to a medium-sized bowl and whisk together. Set mixture aside.

- Add the coconut oil, egg white, and vanilla to a separate medium-sized bowl and whisk together. Stir in the milk and maple syrup.

- Add the flour mixture and stir until the ingredients are completely combined then, add shredded carrot and stir gently.

- Chill the mixture for 30 minutes in the fridge.

- Preheat oven to 325 F and line cookie sheet with parchment paper.

- Use a tablespoon to drop 15 scoops of the mixture onto the cookie sheet. Use a spatula to flatten scoops to your desired thickness and width.

- Bake for 10 - 13 minutes (time depends on the thickness of cookies)

- Cool for 10 minutes then serve.

Note: Any milk will work in place of nonfat milk.

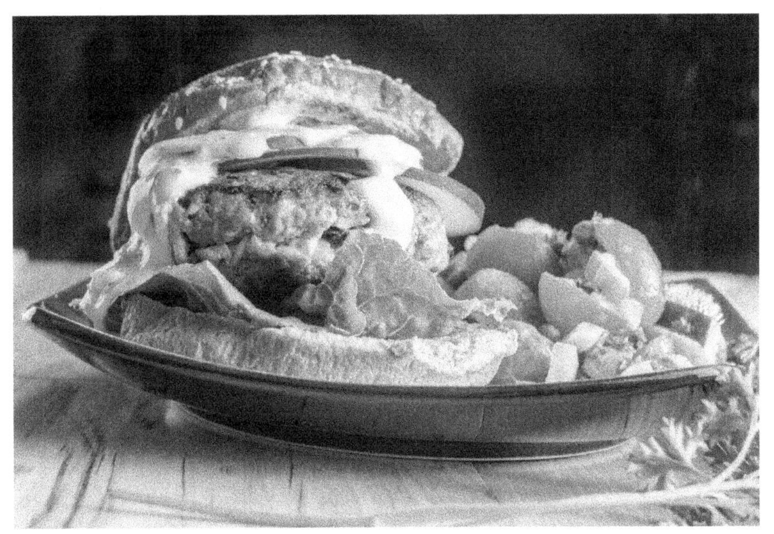

Lunch Recipes

Avocado & Cucumber Sandwich

This scrumptious avocado and cucumber sandwich is loaded with anti-inflammatory ingredients and is so good! Quick, easy, and super healthy!

Anti-Inflammatory Ingredients: lemon juice, pepper, cucumber, red bell pepper, and avocado

Servings: 1
Time: 10 minutes

Ingredients

2 slices mozzarella cheese
2 tsp lemon juice
Pinch of salt
Ground pepper to taste

2 slices whole wheat sandwich bread,
lightly toasted
⅓ cup thinly sliced cucumber
¼ cup thinly sliced red bell pepper
⅓ avocado, sliced

Instructions

Stir lemon juice, salt, and pepper together
in a small bowl. Put a slice

of mozzarella cheese on each slice of
whole wheat bread. Spread half the
mixture on each slice of toast. Layer one
slice with cucumber, pepper, and avocado,
then top with the other slice and serve.
Enjoy!

Pasta Salad With Walnuts & Feta

This hearty Whole Wheat Pasta Salad has nine anti-inflammatory ingredients and is so yummy! Have it as a main course or as a side dish. It's also great for bar-b-ques, picnics, or any potluck - it is sure to be a winner.

Anti-Inflammatory Ingredients: tomatoes, basil, walnuts, extra virgin olive oil, onion, spinach, garlic, pepper

Servings: 8
Time: 1 hour

Ingredients

1 pound whole-wheat pasta

½ lb ripe tomatoes

1 cup finely chopped fresh basil leaves

½ cup chopped walnuts

2 Tbsp extra virgin olive oil

¾ cup crumbled feta cheese

½ cup diced red onion

1 cup finely chopped baby spinach leaves

2 cloves of garlic, minced

salt & pepper to taste

Instructions

- Cook the pasta according to the directions on the package.
- Meanwhile, rinse, core, seed, and chop tomatoes.
- Add all of the remaining ingredients to a large bowl and blend. Add cooked pasta and mix well. Add salt and pepper to taste and serve.

Hummus Veggie Sandwich

This healthy, hearty, hummus and veggie sandwich is a great way to get your anti-inflammatory veggies in. Avocado, mixed greens, red bell pepper, cucumber, and carrots - oh my!

Anti-Inflammatory Ingredients: avocado, mixed greens, red bell pepper, cucumber, carrot

Servings: 1
Time: 10

Ingredients

2 slices whole-grain bread
3 tablespoons hummus
¼ avocado, mashed
½ cup mixed salad greens
¼ medium red bell pepper, sliced

¼ cup sliced cucumber

¼ cup shredded carrot

Instructions

- Spread one slice of bread with hummus and the other with avocado. Fill the sandwich with greens, bell pepper, cucumber, and carrot. Slice in half and serve.

Artichoke Almond Orzo

Let the flavors in this dish take you to Italy with the combination of sun-dried tomatoes, artichoke hearts, and orzo. Delish!

Anti-Inflammatory Ingredients: artichoke, almonds, sun-dried tomatoes, basil, pepper, extra virgin olive oil

Servings: 2
Time: 25 minutes

Ingredients

½ cup whole wheat orzo

1 cup vegetable broth

6 artichoke hearts (canned, quartered)

1 ½ Tbsp Almonds (slivered)

2 Tbsp Sun-dried tomatoes (chopped)

2 Tbsp Parmesan Cheese (grated)

½ tsp dried basil

Salt and pepper (to taste)

1 tsp extra virgin olive oil

Instructions

- Bring the broth and the orzo to a boil.
- Lower heat to medium and cook until the broth is absorbed, about 20 minutes, stirring frequently.
- Stir in the remaining ingredients and serve.

Greek Chicken Wrap

This Greek Chicken Wrap is loaded with anti-inflammatory ingredients and is really good! It is the perfect meal to make ahead of time and take on the go.

Anti-Inflammatory Ingredients: extra virgin olive oil, oregano, garlic, lettuce, tomatoes, onion, cucumber, and olives

Servings: 4
Time: 45 minutes

Ingredients

2 bone-in chicken breasts
1½ tsp extra virgin olive oil
Pinch of dried oregano
Pinch of garlic powder
Pinch lemon pepper
4 cups romaine, chopped
⅓ cup cherry tomatoes, sliced
¼ cup red onion

½ cup cucumber, chopprd

4 Tbsp kalamata olives

½ cup feta cheese

1 Tbsp red wine vinegar

1 Tbsp olive oil

Fresh lemon wedges (optional)

4 large whole wheat wraps

½ cup prepared hummus

Instructions

- Preheat oven to 375 degrees.
- Line a baking sheet with foil and spray with cooking spray.
- Place 2 chicken breasts on baking sheet, season with salt, pepper, dried oregano, and lemon pepper.
- Drizzle with 1 ½ teaspoons of olive oil and bake for 35-40 minutes or until chicken is cooked through.
- Place chopped romaine in a bowl.
- Top with cherry tomatoes, red onion, cucumbers, olives, and feta cheese.

- Sprinkle with a few shakes of dried oregano.
- To dress, drizzle with vinegar and olive oil. Squeeze fresh lemon juice over it all (1 large wedge is fine). Stir and adjust seasonings if necessary.

Wrap Instructions: spread 2 tablespoons of hummus on whole wheat wrap. Top with slices of chicken, and a portion of Greek salad. Roll, wrap and enjoy!

Sweet Potato
Herb Fries

These Sweet Potato Fries are sure to become a favorite. They are cheesy, flavorful, and crisp. Yum!

Anti-Inflammatory Ingredients: sweet potatoes, parsley, chives, extra virgin olive oil, garlic, pepper

Servings: 3
Time: 45 minutes

Ingredients

3 sweet potatoes
1 Tbsp parsley chopped fine
1 Tbsp chives chopped fine
1 Tbsp parmesan cheese
2 Tbsp extra virgin olive oil

1 Tbsp minced garlic

salt & pepper to taste

Instructions

- Preheat oven to 450 degrees.
- Wash the sweet potatoes leaving the skin on, and slice them the length of the potato.
- Mix the olive oil, garlic, salt, and pepper in a bowl and toss the potatoes to coat them.
- Place them on a cooking sheet and bake for 30 minutes.
- After they're done, sprinkle with parsley, chives, and parmesan cheese. Enjoy! They make a great healthy snack or even lunch (I have them as a meal).

Spicy Black Bean Burgers

One bite of these spicy black bean burgers and you'll be hooked. You're gonna love them! They are loaded with super healthy anti-inflammatory ingredients and are so good.

Anti-Inflammatory Ingredients: extra virgin olive oil, onion, garlic, carrot, red bell pepper, black beans, nuts, cayenne pepper, black pepper, avocado

Servings: 4
Time: 1 hour

Ingredients

1 tablespoon extra virgin olive oil

1 small onion, finely chopped

1 clove garlic, finely minced

½ cup shredded carrot

½ cup red bell pepper chopped

2 cans organic black beans, well rinsed

½ cup toasted nuts (your choice)

2 eggs

½ cup breadcrumbs

1 tbsp cumin

1 tsp cayenne pepper

1 tbsp hot sauce

Freshly ground salt & black pepper to taste

1 avocado, peeled, & sliced

whole wheat hamburger buns

Instructions

- Preheat the oven to 350° F and line a large baking sheet with parchment paper.
- In a large skillet, heat the olive oil over medium heat. Add onion, garlic, carrot, and bell pepper, and sauté, stirring occasionally, until vegetables are soft and onion is translucent, about 6-8 minutes.
- Drain one of the cans of black beans, rinse well, and place into the bowl of a food processor. Add nuts and sautéed vegetables. Process until the mixture resembles a paste.
- Drain the remaining can of beans, rinse well, and place into a large glass mixing bowl; mash lightly with a potato masher.
- Add pureed bean mixture and stir to combine. Then add eggs, bread

crumbs, and seasoning. Stir well to combine.

- Using a ½ cup measuring cup, dip into bean mixture and mound onto the prepared baking sheet, pressing lightly to flatten. Leave space between the mounds.

- Bake in preheated oven until completely dry and somewhat crisp; it takes around 45 minutes. Place burgers on whole wheat buns and serve with sliced avocado.

Mediterranean Pasta Salad

This Mediterranean pasta salad is so refreshing! It's one of those dishes that will have everyone asking for the recipe - and so easy to make. It is also the perfect dish to make on a Sunday for healthy lunches throughout the week.

Anti-Inflammatory Ingredients: extra virgin olive oil, lemon juice, garlic, pepper, tomatoes, bell pepper, cucumber, red onion, and black olives

Ingredients

16 oz or 1 lb whole wheat or multigrain Orzo
1 Tbsp Extra Virgin Olive Oil
3 Tbsp Lemon Juice
3 Tbsp Minced garlic

Italian seasoning (to taste)

Salt and pepper (to taste)

10 Cherry Tomatoes (halved)

1 oz Feta Cheese crumbles or Provolone, cubed

1 Green Bell Pepper (chopped)

1 Cucumber (chopped)

¼ cup Red Onion

4 Tbsp Black Olives (drained, sliced)

Instructions

- Prepare orzo according to package directions.
- Drain and rinse in cold water to stop cooking; drain again.
- Set aside to cool.
- Meanwhile whisk the extra virgin olive oil, lemon juice, garlic, Italian seasoning, salt, and pepper together in a small bowl. (If you like a lot of

dressing add 1 tablespoon of water and more lemon juice.)

- In a large bowl combine pasta with tomatoes, cheese, green pepper, olives, and pimentos.
- Pour in olive oil dressing and toss to coat.

Easy Salmon Cakes

These salmon cakes are perfect for lunch or dinner. They are light, super healthy, and loaded with anti-inflammatory goodness!

Anti-Inflammatory Ingredients: salmon, extra virgin olive oil, pepper, lemon, celery, onion, garlic, basil

Servings: 10
Time: 40 minutes

Ingredients

3 filets 4 oz wild salmon (fresh or frozen)
drizzle extra virgin olive oil
salt and pepper to taste
juice of ½ a lemon
2 ribs celery, diced
½ small white onion, diced

2 eggs, whisked

2 Tbsp coconut flour

1 tsp garlic powder

1 tsp salt

½ tsp pepper

½ tsp dried basil

pinch red pepper flake

2 Tbsp coconut oil

Instructions

- Preheat your oven to 350 F and place salmon filets skin down onto a baking sheet and drizzle with olive oil and season with salt and pepper.

- Roast in the oven for 15 -18 minutes (until cooked) then remove skin and set aside.

- Add the salmon filets, lemon juice, seasoning, celery, onion, eggs, and coconut flour to a food processor. Pulse until combined (don't overdo it - just combine the ingredients).

- Using a ⅓ measuring cup, scoop the salmon mixture into the cup and press down with your hands, then place the patty onto a plate and repeat for the rest of the salmon.

- Heat a large skillet on medium-high heat. Add the coconut oil and allow it to get warm (test the oil by sprinkling a drop of water into the pan and seeing if the oil sizzles immediately - if it does, it's ready).

- Place 4 - 5 salmon patties (or however many will fit into your pan) and cook for 3-4 minutes, then remove. Garnish with parsley.

Note: If you don't own a food processor, use canned salmon in place of the fresh or frozen.

Greek Chicken Burgers

These Greek Chicken Burgers are perfect for grill outs but can also be made in the oven. This is one of those recipes that you will make over and over again. It is delicious and loaded with nine anti-inflammatory ingredients!

Anti-Inflammatory Ingredients: red onion, garlic, parsley, oregano, pepper, extra virgin olive oil, cucumber, lemon juice, and parsley

Servings: 4
Time: 30 minutes

Ingredients

1 lb Ground chicken

1 Red onion minced

1 Egg

2 Cloves of garlic minced

¾ cup of whole wheat bread crumbs

½ cup of fresh parsley chopped

½ tsp of dried oregano

Salt and pepper to taste

¼ tsp of red pepper flakes (optional)

1 Tbsp of extra virgin olive oil (if making in a pan)

Greek Sauce Ingredients

1 cup of plain Greek yogurt

1 Tbsp of extra virgin olive oil

½ Cucumber, diced

1 Pinch of garlic powder

2 Tbsp of fresh lemon juice

¼ cup chopped parsley

Salt and pepper to taste

Toppings

4 - 8 lettuce leaves

½ Red onion, sliced

Cucumber slices (desired amount)

2 Tomatoes sliced

4 Whole wheat hamburger buns

Instructions

If you are grilling the burgers, put aluminum foil on the grill and place the patties on top. Follow the directions below just skip the oven. The burgers come out great either way.

Instructions For Burgers

- Heat the olive oil in a medium skillet over medium-high heat. Add the onion to the pan and cook for about 3 minutes, then add the garlic and cook for another minute. Set aside to cool.
- In a large bowl, mix the egg, parsley, oregano, ground chicken, and cooled onion/garlic mixture (add red pepper if you want to use it) mix well.

- Add the salt, pepper, and breadcrumbs, mixing well.
- Preheat your oven to 375 degrees (***skip this step if you are grilling.) and form the mixture into 4 patties of equal size.
- Transfer to a pan and cook in the oven for 30 minutes or until patties are thoroughly cooked.

Greek Sauce

While the burgers are cooking, mix everything except the parsley in a medium-sized bowl. When mixed well, stir in the parsley.

When the Burgers are Cooked

Place each burger on half of the bun. Top with ¼ cup of Greek sauce, tomato slices,

and lettuce leaves. Put the top half of the
bun on the burger and serve with other
condiments if desired.

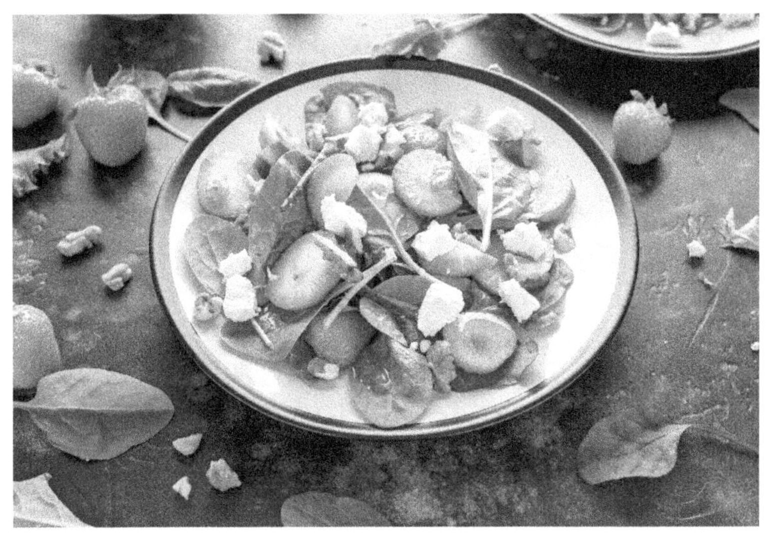

Salad Recipes

Strawberry Spinach Salad

This beautiful and refreshing spinach salad is a delight! The combination of these ingredients come together beautifully. I could eat this salad every day and never get tired of it - it is so good!

Anti-Inflammatory Ingredients: spinach, strawberries, walnuts, garlic, extra virgin olive oil, pepper, red onion, and black pepper

Servings: 4
Time: 20 minutes

Salad Ingredients

4 cups spinach

1 lb strawberries

1 small red onion

3 Tbsp feta cheese

½ cup walnuts

Dressing Ingredients

2 Tbsp extra virgin olive oil
2 tsp balsamic vinegar

1 tsp honey
Pinch of black pepper
1 tsp Dijon mustard

Instructions

- Combine the ingredients for the balsamic vinaigrette in a small bowl. Whisk or stir until the ingredients are mixed well. Set aside.
- Wash the spinach.
- Wash and thinly slice the red onion and strawberries.
- Roughly chop or break the walnuts.
- Combine crumbled feta cheese, spinach, onion, strawberries, and walnuts in a bowl.

- Pour the dressing over the salad and toss well to mix. Serve the salad immediately.

Greek Salad

This traditional Greek salad is delicious! Take a look at all of the anti-inflammatory ingredients!

Anti-Inflammatory Ingredients: oregano, olive oil, garlic, black pepper, onion, tomato, cucumber, bell pepper, basil, olives, parsley

Servings: 4
Time: 15 minutes

Dressing Ingredients

1 clove garlic, grated or pressed
1 tsp dried oregano
¼ cup fresh lemon juice, strained of seeds & pulp
½ cup extra virgin olive oil

½ tsp salt

¼ tsp freshly ground black pepper

Salad Ingredients

2 tsp salt

1 medium red onion, halved and thinly sliced   3 tomatoes, cut into wedges

1 cucumber, peeled and cut into chunks

1 green bell pepper, seeded and sliced

1 red bell pepper, seeded and sliced

¼ cup chopped fresh basil

½ cup pitted and halved Kalamata olives

2 Tbsp fresh Italian parsley

6 ounces feta cheese, sliced

6 lemon wedges

Dressing Instructions

Combine all the ingredients in a jar, shake well and let stand for 30 minutes. Leftover dressing can be stored in the refrigerator for up to 5 days. Makes about 1 ¼ cups.

Salad Instructions

- Combine salt with 2 cups of water in a bowl and add the red onion slices. Let the onions soak for 15 minutes then rinse and drain well.
- In a large bowl toss the tomatoes, cucumbers, and peppers with the basil and enough of the dressing to coat the vegetables well. Adjust the seasonings to taste. Plate in a high mound on a large plate and garnish with olives, parsley, feta, and lemon wedges and serve.

Beet Salad

This Beet Salad is creamy and tangy - a great combination! If you are a beet lover, you are going to love this beet salad recipe.

Anti-Inflammatory Ingredients: beets, walnuts, salad greens, and extra virgin olive oil

Servings: 4
Time: 40 minutes

Ingredients

4 medium beets - scrubbed, trimmed, and cut in halves
⅓ cup chopped walnuts
3 Tbsp maple syrup
1 (10 oz) package mixed baby salad greens
½ cup 100% real orange juice

¼ cup balsamic vinegar

½ cup extra-virgin olive oil

2 oz goat cheese

Instructions

- Place beets into a saucepan, and fill with enough water to cover. Bring to a boil, then cook for 20 to 30 minutes, until tender. Drain, cool, and then cut into cubes.

- While the beets are cooking, place the walnuts in a skillet over medium-low heat. Heat until warm and starting to toast, then stir in the maple syrup. Cook and stir until evenly coated, then remove from the heat and set aside to cool.

- In a small bowl, whisk together the orange juice concentrate, balsamic vinegar, and olive oil to make the dressing.

- Place equal amounts of baby greens onto each of the four salad plates, divide the candied walnuts equally and sprinkle over the greens. Place equal amounts of beets over the greens, and top with pieces of goat cheese. Drizzle each plate with desired amount of dressing.

Shrimp & Avocado Salad

This shrimp and avocado salad is perfect for lunch or dinner. The combination of shrimp and creamy avocado is so good! This is one of my all-time favorite salads! Enjoy!

Anti-Inflammatory Ingredients: shrimp, avocado, scallions, extra virgin olive oil, lime juice, ginger, red pepper, mixed greens, cilantro

Serving: 6
Time: 20 minutes

Ingredients

1 lb large peeled, deveined cooked shrimp, chopped

3 ripe avocados, cubed

¼ cup thinly sliced scallions

¼ cup extra-virgin olive oil

¼ cup fresh lime juice

1 Tbsp grated fresh ginger

2 tsp granulated sugar

¾ tsp salt

¼ tsp crushed red pepper

12 cups mixed greens or chopped romaine lettuce

Instructions

- In a medium bowl, gently stir shrimp, avocados, and scallions together.
- Whisk oil, lime juice, ginger, sugar, salt, and crushed red pepper in a small bowl to make the dressing.
- Pour the dressing over the shrimp mixture; gently stir to coat well.
- Divide greens among 6 plates; top evenly with the shrimp mixture. Enjoy!

Roasted Vegetable Salad

Healthy and delicious, this Garlic Roasted Vegetable Salad is great for lunch or dinner.

Anti-Inflammatory Ingredients: garlic, extra virgin olive oil, carrots, beets, lemon juice, pumpkin seeds

Servings: 4
Time: 40 minutes

Ingredients

1 head garlic

5 Tbsp extra virgin olive oil

4 carrots scrubbed and peeled

4 beets scrubbed and trimmed

8 oz rainbow or swiss chard

1 Tbsp lemon juice

¼ cup pumpkin seeds

sea salt to taste

black pepper to taste

Instructions

- Preheat the oven to 350 degrees. Trim the top quarter off the head of garlic and drizzle with ½ tablespoon olive oil. Wrap it in foil and set it in a small oven-proof dish. Bake it for 20 minutes. Remove it from the oven and keep it wrapped to cool. It will continue to cook as it cools.

- Leave the oven on at 350 degrees. While the garlic roasts, bring a pot of water to a boil. Blanch the carrots in the boiling water for 2 minutes. Then add the beets and boil for 8 to 10 minutes. Remove them from the pot of water and run them under cold water. At this point, the skins should easily peel off the beets. Use a peeler if needed for tougher skins.

- Halve the carrots and quarter the beets. Arrange them on a baking sheet. Drizzle with 1 tablespoon of olive oil and sprinkle with salt. Roast for 20 minutes, flipping vegetables halfway through.

- Arrange the chard on another baking sheet. Drizzle with ½ tablespoon oil and a pinch of salt, and rub it all over the leaves. Roast for 5 minutes, or just until the leaves have softened and become slightly browned.

- Next, make the dressing. Squeeze the roasted garlic out of its skin and into a small mixing bowl. Mix in lemon juice and add a pinch of salt. Next, whisk in the remaining 3 tablespoons of olive oil and combine until smooth.

- Lastly, toast the pumpkin seeds in a small skillet over medium heat. Cook, while flipping almost constantly for 2 minutes. Sprinkle with salt.

- To serve, toss the carrots and beets with the garlic dressing. On a large platter, layer roasted chard on the bottom, then the carrots and beets, drizzle more garlic dressing then sprinkle on the pumpkin seeds, black pepper, and more salt if desired.

Delizioso Italian Chicken Salad

This Delizioso Italian Chicken Salad is highly nutritious, anti-inflammatory, super flavorful, and so easy to make. Buon appetito!

Anti-Inflammatory Ingredients: extra virgin olive oil, garlic, pepper, basil, lettuce, tomato, bell pepper, onion

Servings: 4
Time: 1 hour

Chicken Ingredients

1 Tbsp extra virgin olive oil
1 Tbsp Italian seasoning
2 cloves garlic minced
½ tsp fine sea salt

½ tsp ground pepper

1 pinch red pepper flakes

1 lb boneless skinless chicken breast

Salad Dressing Ingredients

1 ½ Tbsp extra-virgin olive oil

2 tsp apple cider vinegar

¼ cup orange juice freshly squeezed

2 Tbsp fresh basil finely chopped

1 tsp Italian seasoning

½ tsp Kosher salt or fine sea salt

Salad Ingredients

3-4 cups chopped romaine lettuce

1 cup chopped tomatoes

½ cup roasted red peppers chopped

½ cup red onion sliced thin

Instructions

- Combine all the chicken ingredients in a medium-sized bowl and marinate in the refrigerator for at least half an hour or up to 4 hours.

- In a separate bowl, combine and whisk all the salad dressing ingredients. Set aside.

- Mix all the salad ingredients into another bowl and set aside.

- Heat a grill pan to medium-high heat and cook chicken for about 4 - 6 minutes per side or until the internal temperature reaches 165° F. Let the chicken sit for 5 minutes, then slice it into bite-sized pieces.

- Drizzle the dressing on salad and toss to combine. Then, place the cooked chicken on top of the salad and serve immediately.

Notes: You can multiply the salad dressing recipe and make it ahead of time. Store it in the refrigerator. It would retain its freshness for 1 to 2 weeks.

Green Goodness Salad

This refreshing Green Goodness Salad is loaded with 10 anti-inflammatory ingredients! Enjoy the benefits of this salad from the inside out as it provides a ton of nutrients that will help keep your skin nourished, hydrated, and glowing. Enjoy!

Anti-Inflammatory Ingredients: cabbage, cucumber, chives, scallions, lemon, extra virgin olive oil, garlic, shallot, walnuts, spinach

Servings: 4
Time: 30 minutes

Ingredients For Salad

Small head green cabbage, finely diced
3 - 4 cucumbers, diced

¼ cup chives, finely sliced

1 bundle scallions, finely sliced

Dressing Ingredients

Juice of 2 lemons

¼ cup of extra virgin olive oil

2 tbsp rice vinegar

2 cloves garlic, minced

1 small shallot, finely sliced or minced

⅓ cup chives, finely sliced

¼ cup walnuts

1 cup fresh basil leaf

1 cup fresh spinach

⅓ cup nutritional yeast

1 tsp salt

Instructions

- Place all salad ingredients into a big bowl. Add all dressing ingredients to a blender and blend until smooth.
- Pour the desired amount of dressing over each salad, toss well, and enjoy!

Salmon Salad

This salmon salad recipe is loaded with 13 anti-inflammatory ingredients. It's super flavorful and so healthy!

Anti-Inflammatory Ingredients: spinach, tomatoes, avocado, cucumber, red onion, extra virgin olive oil, and salmon

Servings: 2
Time: 30 minutes

Ingredients

4 cups of baby spinach
2 tomatoes, chopped
1 avocado, diced
1 cucumber, peeled and sliced
¼ cup red onion, chopped
2 Tbsp extra virgin olive oil

2 salmon filets

Salt and pepper, to taste

Dressing Ingredients

Juice of 2 large lemons, strained

1.5 cups extra-virgin olive oil

1 Tbsp Italian seasoning

1 tsp dried dill

1.5 tsp Sea Salt

1.5 tsp Black pepper

2 Tbsp minced garlic

Instructions

- Season the salmon filets and put aside. Heat extra virgin olive oil in a large non-stick saute pan over medium heat. Add the salmon, skin side down and cook for 10 minutes.

- Turn the salmon over and cook for another 5 minutes or until thoroughly cooked.

- Separate the salad ingredients into two bowls.
- Whisk the salad dressing ingredients together and pour the desired amount over each salad.
- Top each salad bowl with a salmon filet.

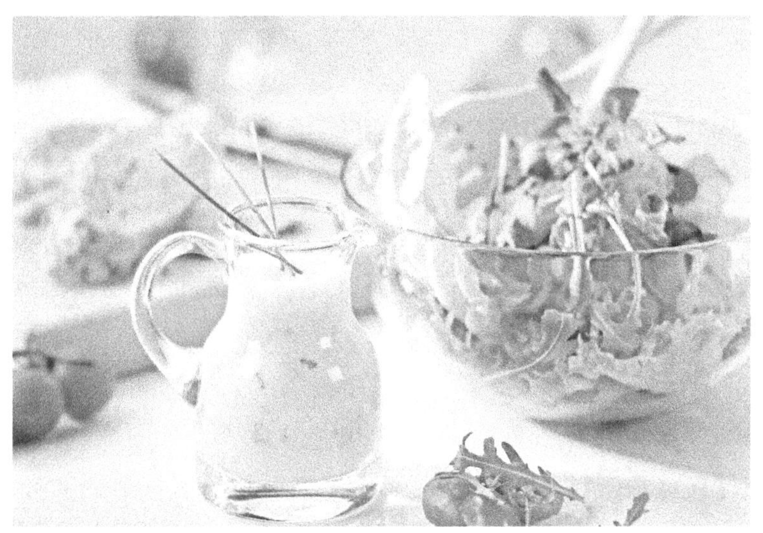

Salad Dressing Recipes

Homemade Ranch Salad Dressing

Anti-Inflammatory Ingredients: lemon, garlic, onion, parsley, dill chives, and black pepper

Servings: 4
Time: 10 minutes

Ingredients

½ cup plain Greek yogurt

1 ½ tsp lemon juice

2 Tbsp water

1 tsp garlic powder

1 Tbsp fresh parsley

¼ tsp onion powder

½ tsp dried dill

½ tsp dried or fresh chives

¼ tsp salt (more to taste if needed)

Dash of pepper

Instructions

- Add all ingredients to a medium size bowl.
- Mix well until ingredients are all combined, and mixture is smooth. If you'd like it to be a little thinner, just add a little bit of water until it reaches desired consistency. You can also mix ingredients in a blender if you prefer.

Garlicky Dill
Salad Dressing

Anti-inflammatory Ingredients: lemon, extra-virgin olive oil, dill, black pepper, and garlic

Servings: 6
Time: 10 minutes

Ingredients

Juice of 2 large organic lemons, remove seeds and strain

1.5 cups extra-virgin olive oil

1 Tbsp organic Italian seasoning

1 tsp dried dill organic

1.5 tsp Sea Salt

1.5 tsp Black pepper

2 Tbsp garlic minced

Instructions

- Combine all ingredients in a glass jar or bottle with a lid. Shake it to mix all of the ingredients well before each use.
- Leftover salad dressing can be refrigerated for later use and should be used within one week.

Creamy Mediterranean Salad Dressing

Anti-inflammatory Ingredients: basil, parsley, green onion, garlic, lemon, extra virgin olive oil, black pepper, and cayenne pepper

Servings: 8
Time: 10 minutes

Instructions

1 cup fresh basil, chopped

1 cup fresh flat leaf parsley, chopped

¼ cup diced green onion

1 clove garlic, minced

1 tsp apple cider vinegar

2 Tbsp fresh squeezed lemon juice

¼ cup extra virgin olive oil

1 cup plain Greek yogurt

⅛ tsp sea salt

⅛ tsp black pepper

⅛ tsp cayenne pepper

Instructions

In a food processor, process all ingredients on high until completely pureed, about 1 minute. Make sure there are no lumps.

Any left over dressings can be stored in the refrigerator for up to 5 days.

Enjoy!

Balsamic Vinaigrette

Anti-Inflammatory Ingredients: garlic, black pepper, and extra virgin olive oil

Servings: 6
Time: 10 minutes

Ingredients

½ cup balsamic vinegar

2 tsp raw honey or maple syrup

2 garlic cloves, grated

2 tsp Dijon mustard

½ tsp sea salt

½ tsp ground black pepper

1 cup extra-virgin olive oil

Instructions

- Whisk together the vinegar, honey, garlic, mustard, salt, and several grinds of pepper in a small bowl.

- Add the olive oil while whisking and continue to whisk until the dressing is emulsified. You can also combine everything in a jar with a tight-fitting lid and shake until thoroughly combined.

Italian Salad Dressing

Anti-Inflammatory Ingredients: extra virgin olive oil, lemon juice, parsley, oregano, thyme, and black pepper

Servings: 6 servings
Time: 10 minutes

Ingredients

¼ cup extra virgin olive oil

2 Tbsp white wine vinegar

2 Tbsp lemon juice

1 Tbsp finely chopped fresh parsley

1 tsp honey

1 tsp dried oregano

1 garlic clove, grated

½ tsp Dijon mustard

½ tsp thyme

¼ tsp sea salt

¼ tsp fresh ground black pepper

2 Tbsp parmesan cheese, optional

Instructions

- Whisk oil, vinegar, lemon juice, parsley, honey, oregano, garlic, mustard, thyme, salt, and pepper in a medium size bowl.
- Stir in the parmesan cheese

Mexican Ranch Salad Dressing

Anti-Inflammatory Ingredients: avocado, lemon juice, extra virgin olive oil, garlic, parsley, dill, and black pepper

Servings: 4
Time: 10 minutes

Ingredients

1 medium avocado

½ cup unsweetened almond milk

2 Tbsp lemon juice

½ Tbsp extra virgin olive oil

1 garlic clove

1 tsp garlic powder

1 tsp onion powder

1 tsp dried parsley

1 tsp dried dill

1 tsp of dijon or stone ground mustard

1 tsp maple syrup

2 Tbsp fresh parsley

½ tsp ground black pepper

½ tsp sea salt

Instructions

- Add all ingredients to a blender and process until smooth.
- If the dressing is thicker than you'd like, just add a little more unsweetened almond milk until it reaches your desired consistency.
- Pour the dressing into a serving container, jar, or bottle. Refrigerate any leftover dressing and use within 2 - 3 days.

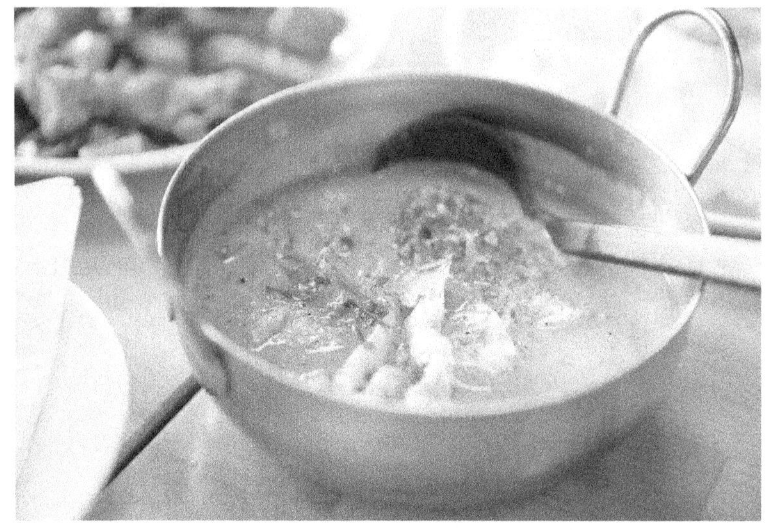

Soup Recipes

Vegetable Soup

This immune-boosting Vegetable Soup is rich and creamy. Freeze some to have on hand for the next time you are feeling under the weather. It's really good, so good for you, and packed with 11 anti-inflammatory ingredients.

Anti-Inflammatory Ingredients: extra virgin olive oil, onion, garlic, ginger, turmeric, cumin, cayenne pepper, carrots, sweet potato, lemon juice, and green onions

Servings: 4
Time: 45 minutes

Ingredients

1 tsp extra virgin olive oil

1 small white onion, chopped

2 cloves garlic, minced

1-inch of ginger, peeled and minced

½ tsp ground turmeric

½ tsp ground cumin

⅛ tsp cayenne pepper (optional)

2 large organic carrots, chopped

1 cup frozen sweet potato chunks

32 oz vegetable broth

2 Tbsp fresh lemon juice

¼ cup nonfat plain yogurt

1 Tbsp chopped green onions

Instructions

In a large soup pot, heat olive oil over medium-low heat. Cook onions until soft and translucent. Add garlic and ginger - cook, until golden and fragrant, less than one minute. Add turmeric, cumin, and cayenne (optional) and stir to combine.

Add carrots and potato chunks to the pot. Pour in vegetable broth and bring to a simmer. Cover and cook for 25-30 minutes, or until soft. Use a blender to puree the soup until smooth. Stir in lemon juice.

Top with yogurt and onions. Sprinkle with more cayenne (optional). Enjoy!

Lemon Chicken Orzo Soup

This super healthy Lemon Chicken Orzo Soup is loaded with 9 anti-inflammatory ingredients. It is super easy to make and delish!

Anti-Inflammatory Ingredients: extra virgin olive oil, oregano, black pepper, onion, carrots, celery, garlic, kale, and lemon juice

Servings: 6
Time: 40 minutes

Ingredients

2 Tbsp extra-virgin olive oil, divided
1 lb boneless, chicken breasts, cut into
1-inch pieces
1 tsp dried oregano
1¼ tsp salt, divided

¾ tsp ground pepper, divided

2 cups chopped onions

1 cup chopped carrots

1 cup chopped celery

2 cloves garlic, minced

1 bay leaf

4 cups unsalted chicken broth

⅔ cup orzo pasta, preferably whole-wheat

4 cups chopped kale

1 lemon, zested and juiced

Instructions

- Heat 1 tablespoon extra virgin olive oil in a large pot over medium heat. Add chicken and sprinkle with ½ teaspoon oregano (and/or thyme), salt, and pepper. Cook, stirring occasionally until lightly browned, 5 minutes. Then transfer the chicken to a plate.

- Add the remaining 1 tablespoon extra virgin olive oil, onions, carrots, and celery to the pot. Cook until the vegetables are soft and lightly browned, 5 minutes. Add garlic, bay leaf, and the remaining ½ teaspoon oregano (and/or thyme). Cook, stirring, until fragrant, about 1 minute.

- Add broth and bring to a boil. Add orzo. Reduce heat to maintain a simmer, cover, and cook for 5 minutes. Add kale and the chicken, along with any accumulated juices. Continue cooking until the orzo is tender and the chicken is cooked through, 8- 10 minutes more.

- Remove from heat. Remove bay leaf. Stir in lemon zest, lemon juice, and the remaining ¾ teaspoon salt and ¼ teaspoon pepper. Enjoy!

Vegetable Chicken Soup

This Vegetable Chicken Soup is spicy and rich with smoky flavors from garlic and roasted poblano pepper. It is delicious and packed with 7 anti-inflammatory ingredients. Enjoy!

Anti-Inflammatory Ingredients: poblano peppers, onion, bell pepper, garlic, beans, tomatoes, and spinach

Servings: 8
Time: 1 hour

Ingredients

2 medium poblano peppers
2 tsp canola oil
12 oz boneless, chicken breast, shredded
1 onion, chopped
1 large red bell pepper
1½ cups green beans

4 cloves garlic, minced

1 Tbsp chili powder

1½ tsp ground cumin

6 cups reduced-sodium chicken broth

1 (15 oz) can black beans or pinto beans

1 (14 oz) can diced tomatoes

4 cups chopped chard or spinach

1½ cups corn kernels, fresh or frozen

½ cup chopped fresh cilantro

½ cup fresh lime juice

lime wedges for serving

Instructions

To roast poblanos, place oven rack about 5 inches from the heat source; and then preheat broiler

Line the broiler pan with foil. Broil whole poblanos, turning once, until starting to blacken, about 10 minutes. Then remove them and set aside to cool.

When the poblanos are cool enough to handle, peel, seed, stem, and coarsely chop, set aside.

Heat the oil in a large soup pot or Dutch oven over medium-high heat.

Add the chicken and cook, turning occasionally, until lightly browned, about 5 minutes. Transfer to a plate and set aside.

Reduce the heat to medium and add onion, bell pepper, green beans, and garlic. Cook, stirring, until beginning to soften, 5 to 10 minutes.

Stir in chili powder and cumin and cook, stirring, until fragrant, less than a minute. Stir in broth, beans, tomatoes, and the chopped poblanos; bring to a boil. Reduce heat to maintain a simmer and cook, stirring occasionally, until the vegetables are tender, about 15 minutes.

Add the chicken and juices, chard (or spinach), and corn; return to a simmer and cook for 15 minutes more to heat through and blend flavors. Top each portion with 1 tablespoon each cilantro and lime juice; serve with lime wedges.

Roasted Red Bell Pepper Soup

This creamy, anti-inflammatory Roasted Red Bell Pepper Soup is wonderful! Serve hot with a dollop of sour cream, and/or goat cheese.

Anti-Inflammatory Ingredients: red bell pepper, onion, garlic, extra virgin olive oil, beans, and pepper

Servings: 6
Time: 1 hour

Ingredients

3 red bell peppers
1 onion, chopped
1 Tbsp minced garlic
1 Tbsp extra virgin olive oil
2 (15 oz) cans cannellini beans, drained and rinsed

2 (14.5 oz) can chicken broth

salt and pepper to taste

Topping

Desired amount of sour cream and/or
goat cheese

Instructions

- Preheat oven to broil.
- Place the bell peppers on a baking
  sheet and broil them on the top rack
  of the oven, using tongs to turn them
  as each side blackens. Allow the
  blackened peppers to cool for about
  30 minutes. Then peel the skin off the
  peppers and discard the stem and
  all the seeds. Chop the peppers and
  set aside.
- In a large pot over medium heat,
  saute the onion and garlic in the oil
  for 5 minutes, or until the onion is
  translucent. Now add the chopped,

roasted red bell peppers and saute for 3 more minutes.

- Next, add the chicken broth and the beans, stirring well. Using a blender, puree the soup in small batches and return to the pot over low heat for 5 minutes. Enjoy!

Spicy Black Bean Soup

This Spicy Black Bean Soup is delicious and is an incredibly healthy meal. Another one that I never get tired of. Enjoy!

Anti-Inflammatory Ingredients: extra virgin olive oil, onion, carrot, celery, red bell pepper, oregano, and avocado

Servings: 6
Time: 45 minutes

Ingredients

2 Tbsp extra virgin olive oil

1 onion, chopped

1 carrot, chopped

1 celery stalk, chopped

1 red bell pepper, chopped

1 Tbsp cumin

1 tsp oregano

1 tsp salt

½ tsp pepper

3 cloves garlic, minced

1 (28 oz) canned fire roasted tomatoes

2 chipotle peppers in adobo sauce,
chopped

32 oz vegetable broth

3 cans (15 oz) black beans

1 avocado, sliced

Note: tortilla chips and sliced jalapeño would be great in this spicy black bean soup.

Instructions

- In a large pot, heat oil over medium heat and then add the onion, carrot, and celery and cook until softened, about 5 minutes. Add the garlic, cumin, oregano, salt, and pepper and sauté another minute.

- Stir in the crushed tomatoes, chipotle peppers, vegetable broth, and black beans and bring to a boil
- Reduce to low heat and simmer for 20 minutes.
- Serve with optional toppings, if desired. Enjoy!

Comforting Chicken Rice Soup

This soup is the best comfort food - it's hard to believe it's so healthy but it is! Comforting Chicken and Rice Soup is packed with 9 anti- inflammatory ingredients and it is delicious - enjoy!

Anti-Inflammatory Ingredients: extra virgin olive oil, onion, carrots, celery, garlic, ginger, turmeric, pepper, lemon juice

Servings: 6
Time: 1 hour

Ingredients

2 cups brown rice cooked
2 Tbsp extra virgin olive oil
1 yellow onion, chopped

2 carrots, chopped

2 celery stalks, chopped

3 cloves garlic, minced

1 inch peeled ginger, finely chopped

1 Tbsp turmeric seasoning

1 tsp salt

½ tsp pepper

8 cups chicken stock

3 cups cooked shredded chicken breast

1 Tbsp fresh lemon juice

Instructions

- Cook your rice according to package directions.
- Season the chicken breast to taste, cook, shred, and set aside.
- While the rice and chicken are cooking, chop your onion, carrots, celery, garlic, and ginger.

- Heat the oil in a large stock pot and add the onion, carrots, and celery until softened and starting to brown, about 10 minutes. Then add the garlic and ginger and sauté another 3 minutes.

- Add the chicken stock, fresh thyme, salt, and pepper, and bring to a simmer. Simmer for 15 minutes.

- Stir in the shredded chicken, fresh lemon juice, and cooked rice. Continue to cook for another 5 minutes and serve.

Three Bean Chili

This quick and easy Three Bean Chili can be prepared in 30 minutes. It's perfect for a healthy lunch or dinner. Double the recipe and freeze some for later and you will be so happy you did!

Anti-Inflammatory Ingredients: extra virgin olive oil, onion, garlic, beans, tomatoes, cocoa, pepper, and green onion

Servings: 4
Time: 30 minutes

Ingredients

1 Tbsp extra virgin **olive oil or**
1 large onion, diced
3 cloves garlic, minced
2 jalapenos, seeds removed and diced
3 Tbsp chili seasoning
1 tsp chipotle seasoning

1 can (15 oz) black beans

1 can (15 oz) kidney beans

1 can (15 oz) pinto beans

1 can (28oz) diced tomatoes, with juice

1 Tbsp cocoa (optional)

1 ½ cups water

salt & pepper, to taste

Toppings

Green onions

Sour cream

Lime wedges

Instructions

- In a large pot, heat olive oil over medium heat, saute onion for 7 minutes, or until tender and translucent. Add the garlic, jalapeno, chili, and chipotle powder, and cook for another 2 minutes.

- Add the beans, tomatoes, cocoa powder, and water or broth, bring to a simmer. Boil, reduce heat, cover, and simmer for 20 minutes, stirring occasionally. Add more water as needed.
- Add salt and pepper to taste.
- Serve with sliced green onions, sour cream, and lime wedges.

Homemade Chicken Soup

You don't need to be sick to enjoy this flavorful soup. It is delicious and packed with 9 anti-inflammatory ingredients! Enjoy!

Anti-Inflammatory Ingredients: extra virgin olive oil, carrots, celery, onion, bell pepper, garlic, thyme, black pepper, and cayenne pepper

Servings: 3 - 4
Time: 30 minutes

Ingredients

1 - 2 Tbsp extra virgin olive oil

3 carrots, chopped

3 ribs celery, chopped

½ onion, chopped

½ orange pepper, chopped

½ yellow pepper, chopped

1 quart organic chicken broth

2 cups water

5 cloves garlic, chopped

1.5 lbs cooked chicken breast, shredded

½ cup fresh thyme

½ cup green onions, sliced

Salt and pepper, to taste

Cayenne pepper, to taste

Instructions

- Add olive oil to a large pot over medium heat.
- Chop carrots and add them to the pot.
- Add a few shakes of salt, pepper, and cayenne to the carrots. Stir and let sit while you chop the celery, onion & peppers. Continue to stir the carrots every few minutes.

- Add the onions & celery to the pot, and stir.

- Add the shredded chicken to a bowl and set aside.

- Add the orange & yellow peppers to the pot, and stir to combine. Continue to stir the mixture, cook for a few minutes before moving on to the next step.

- Add the chicken broth & water to the vegetables in the pot.

- Chop the garlic and add to the bowl with the chicken. Add salt, pepper and cayenne pepper into the bowl with the chicken & garlic. Mix all of these ingredients together well.

- Add the chicken mixture to the pot, and stir to combine. Turn up the heat to medium-high and continue to stir for 5 minutes. Reduce heat to simmer and cover. Let it simmer for 5 minutes.

- Chop the green onion and fresh thyme. After a few minutes add the fresh thyme to the pot. Set the chopped green onion aside.
- Stir everything together and turn the heat up to medium-high. Let the soup come to a boil. Once boiling let it continue to boil for 3-5 minutes and be sure to continue to stir.
- Serve with sliced green onion as topping. Enjoy!

Creamy Tomato Basil Soup

I love this Creamy Tomato Basil Soup and always keep some in my freezer for a rainy day. It's simple and easy to make but so good! Enjoy!

Anti-Inflammatory Ingredients: onion, garlic, extra virgin olive oil, tomato, black pepper, basil

Servings: 4
Time: 40 minutes

Ingredients

1 large yellow onion, diced
3 large cloves garlic, minced
¼ cup plus another 2 Tbsp extra-virgin olive oil, divided
2 ½ lb Roma tomatoes

1 tsp kosher salt
Freshly ground black pepper to taste
10 large fresh basil leaves

Instructions

- Dice the yellow onion and mince the garlic cloves if you haven't already.

- Heat ¼ cup extra-virgin olive oil in a medium pot over medium heat until shimmering. Add the onion and garlic and cook until
soft and aromatic, about 10 minutes. Meanwhile, quarter the tomatoes, then cut each piece in half.

- Add the tomatoes to the pot, increase the heat to medium-high, and cook, stirring frequently, until the tomatoes have softened, and broken apart, about 15 minutes. Remove from the heat. Add 1 teaspoon kosher salt, and 10 large basil leaves, season with black pepper. Stir to combine and let sit for 15 minutes to cool before blending.

- Use an immersion or standard blender to purée the soup, slowly drizzling in 2 tablespoons olive oil while blending, until smooth or desired consistency. Taste and season with salt and pepper as needed. Enjoy!

Blending options: An immersion blender is the easiest way to purée this soup, but a standard blender works just as well — and even a food processor can do the trick. If using a blender or a food processor, work in batches if needed and make sure the feed hole or tube is open while blending so that steam can escape — puréeing a hot liquid could result in a messy explosion. **This is why it is important to let it cool a little before blending.**

Carrot Soup

This Carrot Soup is loaded with 8 anti-inflammatory ingredients and is super flavorful. Enjoy!

Anti-Inflammatory Ingredients: extra virgin olive oil, leek, fennel, carrots, butternut squash, garlic, ginger, and turmeric

Servings: 4
Time: 50 minutes

Ingredients

1 Tbsp extra virgin olive oil
1 leek, cleaned and sliced
1 cup chopped fennel (1 small head)
3 cups chopped carrots
1 cup chopped butternut squash
2 garlic cloves, minced

1 Tbsp grated ginger (about 2" piece)
1 Tbsp turmeric powder
Salt & pepper to taste
3 cups vegetable broth
1 can (14.5 oz) coconut milk

Instructions

- Heat the olive oil in a large dutch oven or soup pot. Add the fennel, leeks, carrots, and squash. Saute for 5 minutes or until the veggies start to soften. Add the garlic, ginger, turmeric, salt, and pepper, and saute for a few more minutes.
- Add broth and coconut milk. Bring the mixture to a boil, cover, and simmer for 20 minutes. Let cool before blending.

- Once the soup has cooled, add it to a blender and blend until creamy. You could also use an immersion blender.
- Return soup to pot and simmer for 10 minutes to reheat. Adjust seasonings to taste.
- Serve immediately with a dollop of yogurt and enjoy!

Rosemary & Sweet Potato Soup

This Rosemary and Sweet Potato Soup is a wonderful pairing of ingredients. It's super simple to make, and so good. Enjoy!

Anti-Inflammatory Ingredients: sweet potatoes, garlic, cinnamon, rosemary

Servings: 5
Time: 40 minutes

Ingredients

2 lb sweet potatoes, peeled

2 cups chicken broth

1 tsp garlic powder

1 tsp cinnamon

2 tsp rosemary

Salt and pepper to taste

Instructions

- Place peeled sweet potatoes in a pot and fill with water to cover the potatoes. Bring the water to a boil and cook for about 20 minutes, or until the sweet potatoes are tender. Let cool.
- Place the cooked sweet potatoes and chicken broth in a blender and blend well. Add more broth for desired consistency if needed.
- Add all the spices. Pulse a few more times until the spices are evenly distributed.
- Reheat if needed, and serve. Enjoy!

Roasted Butternut Squash Soup

This easy Roasted Butternut Squash Soup is so cozy and good! Rosemary, sage, and thyme, oh my! Loaded with 10 anti-inflammatory ingredients and ready in just 30 minutes.

Anti-Inflammatory Ingredients: butternut squash, carrots, celery, onion, garlic, sage, thyme, rosemary, cayenne pepper, olive oil

Servings: 8
Time: 1 hour 30 minutes

Ingredients

1 large butternut squash

2 carrots

3 stalks of celery

1 large onion

5 cloves of garlic

6 sage leaves

6 sprigs of thyme

1 sprig of rosemary

¼ tsp cayenne pepper

salt and pepper, to taste

2 Tbsp extra virgin olive oil

3 ½ cups vegetable stock

Instructions

You will need a large baking pan, food processor or blender, large pot, or 4-quart dutch oven.

Peel, pit and chop the butternut squash into 1-inch squares. Chop the carrots, celery, and onions into big chunks. Peel the garlic and cut into halves. Add everything into a baking pan. Add the herbs with stems removed, cayenne pepper, salt, and pepper. Add olive oil and toss to coat.

Roast the vegetable and herb mixture for 1 hour at 350 F or until veggies are soft and tender. To check tenderness, insert a fork into the vegetable. If it comes out easily, then it is done. You will want to check the carrots in particular, as they may take the longest to cook. If the vegetables aren't tender, then cook for another 15 minutes.

Transfer cooked vegetables to a food processor or blender with vegetable stock and puree until smooth and creamy, or until desired consistency is reached. You may need to do this in a couple of batches. You can also blend the soup directly in the pot using an immersion blender.

Pour the mixture into a large pot. Add the remaining vegetable stock and stir well. Cook on medium for 10 minutes. If the consistency of the soup is too thick, just thin it out with some water until you reach your desired consistency.

Top each serving with pumpkin seeds and
a dollop of sour cream (optional) and
serve.

Sweet Potato Lentil Soup

This Moroccan-inspired Sweet Potato Lentil Soup will make your home smell warm and cozy! It's loaded with 11 anti-inflammatory ingredients and is super flavorful. This is a slow cooker recipe but you can cook it on the stovetop if you prefer. You're gonna love it!

Anti-Inflammatory Ingredients: sweet potatoes, carrots, onion, celery, bell pepper, garlic, cumin, cinnamon, turmeric, spinach, and lemon juice

Servings: 6 - 8
Slow Cooker Time: 6 hours

Ingredients

1 lb sweet potatoes, peeled and cubed

1 cup carrots, chopped

1 cup onions, chopped

1 cup celery, chopped

1 red bell pepper, diced

6 cloves garlic, minced or pressed

1 ½ cups green or brown lentils, rinsed

1 ½ tsp coriander

1 ½ tsp cumin powder

1 tsp curry powder

½ tsp smoked paprika

½ tsp ground cinnamon

½ tsp turmeric

⅛ tsp ground nutmeg

6 cups low sodium broth (vegetable or chicken)   2 ½ cups baby spinach, finely chopped

lemon wedges for serving

Instructions

- Place the sweet potatoes, carrots, onions, celery, red bell pepper, garlic, lentils, spices, and 6 cups of broth into a slow cooker. Cover and cook on the low setting for 6-8 hours or on high for 4 - 6 hours. Taste to make sure it's cooked. Then allow to cool before blending.

- Place half the soup into a blender with ½ cup of broth, and blend till smooth.
- Add the puree back into the slow cooker. Stir in the baby spinach and lemon juice. Cover the slow cooker, and cook on low for 30 minutes.
- If needed, you can thin the soup with additional broth to desired consistency.
- Season to taste.
- Serve with warm pita bread.
- Top with whipped greek yogurt and fresh herbs.

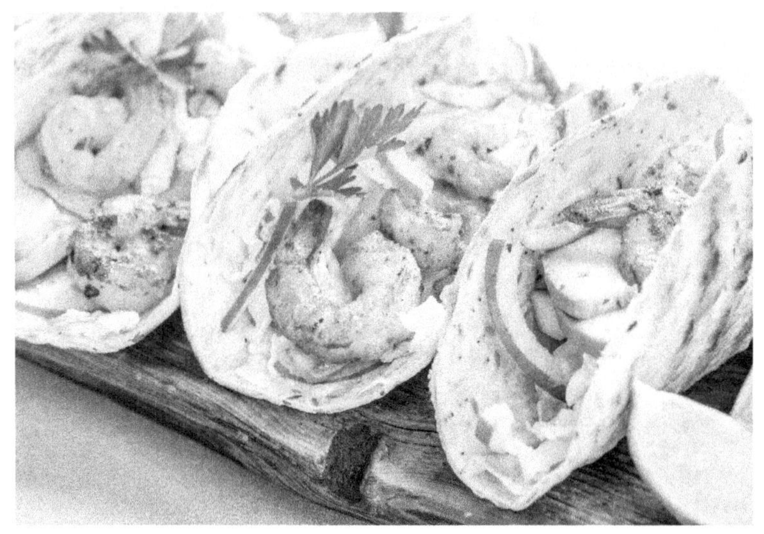

Dinner Recipes

Spinach Pistachio Pesto Pasta

This super flavorful Spinach Pistachio Pesto Pasta can be made in under 30 minutes and is loaded with anti-inflammatory ingredients.

Anti-Inflammatory Ingredients: spinach, basil, pistachios, garlic, lemon juice, black pepper, and extra virgin olive oil

Servings: 8
Time: 30 minutes

Ingredients

1 lb whole grain rigatoni

4 cups packed spinach leaves

2 cups packed basil leaves

¼ cup shelled pistachios

2 cloves garlic

3 Tbsp fresh lemon juice

¼ cup fresh shredded Parmesan cheese

½ tsp salt

¼ tsp black pepper

½ cup extra virgin olive oil

Toppings

Crushed red pepper flakes, to taste
Shredded parmesan cheese, to taste

Instructions

- To cook pasta, follow pasta package instructions.
- To make the pesto, you will need a food processor. Add the spinach, pistachios, basil, garlic, lemon juice, parmesan cheese, olive oil, salt and pepper. Blend until pesto has a smooth consistency.
- Before draining pasta, reserve 1 cup of the pasta water to use later in the recipe then drain pasta.

- Return pasta to pot to add pesto. Add half of the pesto mixture to the pasta and ¼ cup of the pasta water then gently stir to mix. Add remaining pesto and pasta water and stir again until thoroughly mixed.
- Add salt and pepper to taste.
- Top with crushed red pepper flakes and parmesan cheese. Enjoy!

Holy Moly Shrimp Fajitas

These Holy Moly Shrimp Fajitas are delicious! They are loaded with anti-inflammatory ingredients and only take 30 minutes to make. Enjoy!

Anti-Inflammatory Ingredients: oregano, extra virgin olive oil, shrimp, onion, red bell pepper, orange bell pepper, yellow bell pepper, avocado, tomato

Servings: 4
Time: 30 minutes

Ingredients

2 tsp smoked paprika

3 tsp chili powder

2 tsp cumin

1 tsp garlic powder

1 tsp dried oregano

1 tsp salt

1 Tbsp chipotle adobo sauce

2 Tbsp extra virgin olive oil

1 lb shrimp peeled and deveined

1 yellow or red onion halved and sliced

2 red pepper sliced

1 yellow pepper sliced

1 orange pepper sliced

Top with avocado, sour cream, cheese, tomato

Tip: These fajitas are great served with warm whole wheat tortillas.

Instructions

- Preheat the oven 400 F. Add the smoked paprika, chili powder, cumin, garlic powder, oregano, and salt to a medium bowl. Next, add the chipotle in adobo sauce and the olive oil and stir until mixed well.

- Place the shrimp in a medium size bowl and pour half of the spice mixture over the shrimp. Stir well. Cover the shrimp and place in the fridge.

- In a separate bowl, add onion and peppers. Pour the remaining spice mixture over the onion and peppers. Stir well. Spread the onions and peppers evenly onto a large baking sheet. Place in the oven and cook for 20 minutes.

- Remove onions and peppers from the oven and make room on the baking sheet to place the shrimp. Should be shrimp on one side and onions and peppers on the other side separately.

- Add the marinated shrimp to the baking sheet with the onion and peppers in an even layer and bake for 5 - 10 minutes or until the shrimp are pink and have formed a C shape. Serve warm with avocado, tomato, cheese, and sour cream.

Herb Roasted Chicken With Vegetables

This mouth watering Herb Roasted Chicken and Vegetables is infused with flavor and is super easy to make. Not only is it delicious, it has 8 anti-inflammatory ingredients. Enjoy!

Anti-Inflammatory Ingredients: garlic, rosemary, parsley, lemon, extra virgin olive oil, pepper, onion, carrots

Servings: 6
Time: 1 hour 30 minutes

Ingredients

2 cloves garlic, minced
2 Tbsp finely chopped fresh rosemary
2 Tbsp finely chopped fresh parsley

1 lemon, zest and juice

2 Tbsp extra virgin olive oil

1 chicken (4 lb)

Salt and black pepper to taste

1 large russet potato, sliced into

2 onions, quartered

4 large carrots, cut into large chunks

Instructions

- Preheat the oven to 450. Place chicken (breast side up) in a roasting pan deep enough for the vegetables and juice.

- Add the garlic, rosemary, parsley, lemon juice, lemon zest, and olive oil to a medium size bowl. Pour half of the olive oil mixture over the chicken. Spread it over the chicken thoroughly and then season with salt and pepper.

- Mix the potato, onions, and carrots with the remaining olive oil mixture, add a pinch of salt and pepper. Make sure all of the vegetables are coated evenly.

- Place the vegetables in the roasting pan around and underneath the chicken so that the chicken is sitting on the vegetables.

- Cook for 30 minutes, or until the skin has been lightly browned. Reduce the oven temperature to 350 F and cook for another 30 to 45 minutes.

- The chicken is ready when the juices are clear and it has an internal temperature of 165 F.

- Remove the chicken and vegetables from the oven and allow to rest for 10 minutes before serving. Enjoy!

Black Bean & Avocado Burritos

This is one of my favorite meals. It is easy to make and super nutritious. Packed with 7 anti-inflammatory ingredients and yummy - Enjoy!

Anti-Inflammatory Ingredients: extra virgin olive oil, onion, red bell pepper, garlic, black beans, avocado, tomatoes

Servings: 6
Time: 30 minutes

Ingredients

1 Tbsp extra virgin olive oil
½ cup chopped onion
½ cup chopped red bell pepper
1 garlic clove minced
1 can black beans drained

½ tsp cumin

½ tsp paprika

½ tsp chili powder

¼ tsp garlic powder

¼ tsp cayenne pepper

¼ tsp salt

1 avocado pitted and sliced

1 small tomato chopped

2 Tbsp chopped cilantro (optional)

6 medium whole wheat tortillas

1 cup of Monterey Jack cheese

¼ cup sour cream

Chipotle salsa (optional)

Instructions

- Heat the oven to 300. Wrap your tortillas in aluminum foil and place in the oven for 10 - 15 minutes, until thoroughly heated.
- Heat oil in a large pan over medium / high heat. Add onion, bell pepper, and garlic. Cook for 2-3 minutes or

until onion is lightly golden. Add the black beans and seasoning. Cook for another 2-3 minutes. Remove from heat for a few minutes before assembling.

- To assemble, lay the heated tortillas flat, add the black bean mixture, and top with cheese, avocado, salsa, cilantro (optional) and sour cream. Enjoy - I love these!

Marinara & Feta Pasta

Easy, quick, and delicious! I make this recipe every month and never get tired of it. It has 7 anti-inflammatory ingredients and it is so good! I hope you enjoy it as much as I do.

Anti-Inflammatory Ingredients: tomatoes, garlic, extra virgin olive oil, black pepper, basil, walnuts, olives

Servings: 4
Time: 30 minutes

Ingredients

8 oz of whole wheat pasta (fusilli, bow-tie, or penne)
1 ½ cups cherry tomatoes cut in half
2 cloves of garlic minced

1 Tbsp extra virgin olive oil

Black pepper to taste

¼ tsp red pepper flakes

6 basil leave finely chopped

⅓ cup walnut pieces

12 kalamata olives sliced

2 oz crumbled feta

Instructions

Tip: If you want a faster, easier cooking option for this recipe you can use 24 oz of your favorite healthy tomato based pasta sauce. Make sure to check the ingredients!

- Prepare all ingredients so they are ready to use. Slice the tomatoes in half, mince garlic, mince basil, measure out walnuts, slice olives, and dice feta. Set aside.

- Bring a large pot of water to a boil and cook pasta according to package directions.

- While the pasta is cooking, add one tablespoon of olive oil to a large saute pan over medium heat. Saute minced garlic. Add chopped tomatoes, black pepper, and red pepper flakes and saute over medium heat for 5 minutes or until cherry tomatoes are soft and wilted and have begun to release their juices. Remove pan from heat. Before draining pasta, reserve ¼ cup of pasta water.

- Drain pasta, add it to the large saute pan with cherry tomatoes. Add basil, walnuts, olives and most of the feta to the pan. Toss gently to combine. If the pasta seems dry, add a little pasta water to create a sauce.

- Sprinkle the remaining feta on top of the pasta and serve. Enjoy!

Lemon Herb Salmon With Orzo

This Lemon Herb Salmon with Orzo is ready in just 25 minutes! It is really good and has 7 anti-inflammatory ingredients.

Anti-Inflammatory Ingredients: broccoli, extra virgin olive oil, salmon, pepper, chives, parsley, lemon

Servings: 4
Time: 25 minutes

Ingredients

1 cup whole-wheat orzo
2 cups chopped broccoli
4 Tbsp extra-virgin olive oil
1¼ lb skin-on salmon filet, cut into 4 portions
½ tsp salt
½ tsp ground pepper

3 Tbsp chopped fresh dill

1 Tbsp parsley

2 tsp lemon zest

1 Tbsp lemon juice

Instructions

- Cook orzo according to package directions, adding broccoli for the last minute of cooking. Drain and rinse with cold water.
- Heat 1 tablespoon extra virgin olive oil in a large nonstick skillet over medium heat.
- Sprinkle each piece of salmon with ¼ teaspoon salt and pepper.
- Put salmon in the heated skillet skin-side up, and cook until golden brown, 3 to 5 minutes. Flip and cook until the flesh is opaque, 3 to 5 minutes, depending on thickness.

- Whisk 2 tablespoons extra virgin olive oil, herbs, lemon zest, lemon juice and the remaining ¼ teaspoon each salt and pepper in a medium bowl. Add the orzo and broccoli; stir until combined.
- Serve the salmon over orzo mixture. Enjoy!

Fish Tacos

These quick-and-easy Fish Tacos are served with avocado slices and are ready to serve in just 25 minutes. This dish is perfect for a casual weeknight dinner. Delish!

Anti-Inflammatory Ingredients: avocado oil, mahi mahi, avocado, and cabbage

Servings: 4
Time: 25 minutes

Ingredients

1 Tbsp avocado oil
2 tsp no-salt-added Mexican-style seasoning blend
½ tsp salt

1 lb flaky white fish filets, like mahi mahi

1 avocado, sliced

½ cup pico de gallo

8 corn tortillas, warmed

¼ cup cabbage

Instructions

- Preheat oven to 350 F.

- Spray a large rimmed baking sheet with extra virgin olive oil cooking spray.

- Cut the fish into medium size pieces.

- Stir oil, seasoning blend and salt together in a medium bowl. Add fish and toss to coat.

- Transfer to the prepared baking sheet and bake until the fish flakes easily, about 20 minutes, depending on thickness.

- To assemble tacos, place desired amount of fish, 2 slices avocado and

1 tablespoon pico de gallo in each tortilla. Enjoy!

Lemon Chicken & Herb Rice

This Lemon Chicken and Herb Rice recipe is super easy to make. It is Persian-inspired and has a beautiful golden color and a wonderful fragrance. Don't forget the saffron - it makes a big difference.

Anti-Inflammatory Ingredients: extra virgin olive oil, onion, garlic, turmeric, cabbage, lemon, parsley

Servings: 8
Time: 1 hour 30 minutes

Ingredients

2 Tbsp extra virgin olive oil, divided
8 boneless, skinless chicken breast

2 large onions, thinly sliced

½ tsp salt, divided

3 cloves garlic, minced

2 tsp ground turmeric

1 tsp paprika

1 pinch of saffron

3 cups shredded cabbage

4 cups cooked brown rice

¼ cup lemon juice

2 Tbsp chopped fresh Italian parsley

1 lemon, sliced

Instructions

- Preheat oven to 350 degrees F. Coat two 8-inch-square baking dishes or foil pans with extra virgin olive oil cooking spray. Heat 1 tablespoon extra virgin olive oil in a large nonstick skillet over medium heat.

- Add 4 chicken breasts, and cook, turning once, until both sides are lightly browned, 5 - 10 minutes. Transfer the chicken to a plate and set aside. Repeat with the remaining chicken breasts. Pour off all but about 1 tablespoon of fat from the pan.
- Add the remaining 1 tablespoon extra virgin olive oil and onions to the pan and sprinkle with ¼ teaspoon salt. Cook, stirring, until soft and golden, 15 minutes.
- Stir in garlic, turmeric, paprika, and saffron, cook, stirring, for 2 minutes. Transfer the onions to a plate and set aside.
- Return the pan to medium heat and add cabbage. Cook, stirring, until wilted, about 5 minutes. Stir in rice, lemon juice, the remaining ¼

teaspoon salt, and half of the reserved onion. Continue cooking until the rice is well coated and heated through, 5 to 7 minutes.

- Divide the rice mixture between the prepared baking dishes; nestle 4 of the chicken breasts in each dish. Top each with half of the remaining cooked onions. Cover both dishes with foil.
- Bake the remaining casserole, covered, for 30 minutes.
- Uncover and continue baking for another 5 to 10 minutes, until a thermometer inserted in the thickest part of the chicken registers 165 degrees F and the onions are starting to brown around the edges.
- Garnish with parsley and lemon slices. Enjoy!

Cajun Blackened Salmon

This Cajun Blackened Salmon recipe is the best (in my opinion)! The filets of salmon are topped with cajun spices and then cooked to perfection. It is shockingly simple to make and restaurant level delicious!

Anti-Inflammatory Ingredients: salmon, cayenne pepper, oregano, black pepper, thyme, sage, parsley

Servings: 4
Time: 20 minutes

Ingredients

4 (6oz) salmon filet portions skin-on

1 Tbsp paprika

1 tsp sea salt

1 Tbsp onion powder

1 Tbsp garlic powder

1 Tbsp cayenne pepper

¾ Tbsp white pepper

¾ Tbsp black pepper

½ Tbsp dried oregano

½ Tbsp dried sage

2 Tbsp unsalted real butter

2 lemons cut into wedges

½ tsp chopped fresh parsley

Instructions

- Add all spices together in a jar with a lid or small plastic container with a lid and shake until blended well.
- Sprinkle cajun spice liberally over salmon filets on both sides.
- Melt butter in a large saucepan over medium heat until hot.
- Place salmon filets in butter and cook each side 5 - 10 minutes,

depending on the size of the filet. Be sure to cook one side before flipping to blacken properly.

- Squeeze lemon juice on each filet. Sprinkle with parsley and serve. Enjoy!

Side Suggestion: This recipe pairs perfectly with a baked sweet potato as a side dish.

Sweet Potato Tacos

These scrumptious Sweet Potato Tacos are served with a creamy avocado lime dressing. They are loaded with flavorful anti-inflammatory ingredients and are super easy to make. Enjoy!

Anti-Inflammatory Ingredients: sweet potato, extra virgin olive oil, black beans, lime, pepper, avocado, garlic, and scallions

Serves: 2
Time: 30 minutes

Ingredients

1 medium sweet potato, cubed
Extra virgin olive oil for drizzling
½ tsp chili powder

4 whole wheat tortillas

1 cup black beans, cooked

Lime slices, for serving

Sea salt and black pepper, to taste

Avocado dressing:

½ cup whole milk Greek yogurt

1 small avocado

½ garlic clove

Juice of 1 lime

Salt & fresh black pepper, to taste

Toppings

2 scallions, diced

Crumbled feta

Instructions

- Preheat oven to 350° F.
- Line a large baking sheet with parchment paper.

- Toss the sweet potatoes with olive oil, chili powder, salt and pepper, and spread onto the baking sheet. Roast for 30 minutes, or until golden brown.
- Make the avocado yogurt sauce in a small food processor, combine the yogurt, avocado, garlic, lime juice, and a few generous pinches of salt and pepper. Pulse until smooth. Taste and adjust seasonings to desired taste. Chill until ready to use.
- Assemble the tacos with the roasted sweet potatoes, black beans, and avocado dressing, feta cheese, and scallions. Season with salt, pepper, and squeezes of lime. Enjoy!

Three Day Jump Start

Many years ago, I started doing what I call My Three Day Feel Good Diet. Anytime I am feeling run down or depleted, haven't had time to take care of myself properly, or just want to go on a health kick, I do this diet for three days and always feel terrific afterwards. It is super simple, delicious, and does not require a lot of time.

Yes, you are eating the same foods for three days in a row but because the food that you are eating is so good, you will hardly notice and you will feel so good that you won't even care (at least I don't).

In addition to this meal plan, I drink lots of water with lemon, do 30 minutes of yoga, and meditate each day. I do all of these things for three days in a row and it works every single time. I feel great, my skin looks great, and this serves as motivation to continue.

It is a great way to jump start your anti-inflammatory lifestyle. The recipes for all of these meals are located within this book but the specific meal plan is below. I hope that it works as well for you as it has for me!

Three Day Jump Start Meal Plan

Breakfast

Vanilla or plain Greek yogurt, add fresh blueberries and walnuts. Make sure that the yogurt is whole healthy yogurt with no junk ingredients like fructose. Most Greek yogurt is good but make sure to read the list of ingredients.

Lunch

Spinach Salad - Spinach, Strawberries, Red Onions, Feta Cheese, Walnuts, Balsamic Vinaigrette

Dinner

Blackened Salmon with Baked Sweet Potato

Snacks

Dark Chocolate (at least 70%) and Nuts

Conclusion

As with any lifestyle change, you probably will have the most success by starting by slowly. Make slow changes so that they become more doable and more of a lifestyle shift rather than a diet. Try to eat fewer foods that come from packages and eat more that come from the ground - the soil of the earth. Before you know it, you will not even miss the processed foods. Chances are you won't even enjoy the way they taste after you become accustomed to the anti-inflammatory diet/lifestyle. And, before you know it, you'll be reaping the rewards!

Here's to you and your health - Cheers!

Citations

https://www.henryford.com/blog/2020/07/health-benefits-antiinflammatorydiet#:~:text=%E2%80%9CThe%20risk%20of%20heart%20disease,properties%20known%20to%20ease%20inflammation.

https://www.eatingwell.com/article/7894310/anti-inflammatory-meal-plan-for-beginners/

https://www.goodpath.com/learn/anti-inflammatory-diet-meal-plan

https://www.goodpath.com/learn/anti-inflammatory-diet-eat-out

https://fullscript.com/blog/anti-inflammatory-foods

https://www.drweil.com/diet-nutrition/anti-inflammatory-diet-pyramid/dr-weils-anti-inflammatory-food-pyramid/

https://www.healthline.com/nutrition/anti-inflammatory-tea#TOC_TITLE_HDR_6

https://wellbalancedmvmt.com/anti-inflammatory-diet/#:~:text=Listed%20below%20are%20the%20recommended,and%20shellfish%20from%20unpolluted%20waters.

https://www.henryford.com/blog/2020/07/health-benefits-antiinflammatorydiet#:~:text=%E2%80%9CThe%20risk%20of%20heart%20disease,properties%20known%20to%20ease%20inflammation

https://www.health.harvard.edu/staying-healthy/foods-that-fight-inflammation

https://www.webmd.com/diet/what-to-know-about-nightshade-vegetables#:~:text=Nightshade%20is%20a%20family%20of,are%20mainly%20found%20in%20plants.

https://www.medicalnewstoday.com/articles/321745

https://www.eatthis.com/news-proven-ways-to-look-younger-experts/

https://www.healthline.com/nutrition/13-anti-inflammatory-foods#TOC_TITLE_HDR_6

https://www.wellmark.com/blue/nutrition/11-powerhouse-foods-to-soothe-inflammation

https://www.wellandgood.com/inflammation-aging/

https://www.txhealthcare.com/posts/understanding-inflammation/

https://www.webmd.com/diet/health-benefits-rhubarb

https://health.clevelandclinic.org/flaxseed-oil-benefits/

https://www.sciencedirect.com/science/article/pii/S2666354622000114

www.ingramcontent.com/pod-product-compliance
Lightning Source LLC
Chambersburg PA
CBHW061502120726
48001CB00004B/1178